Heraclio Alves Barbosa Junior
Antonio S Guimarães

Orthodontists' Knowledge of Temporomandibular Dysfunction

Heraclio Alves Barbosa Junior
Antonio S Guimarães

Orthodontists' Knowledge of Temporomandibular Dysfunction

Research carried out in the State of Amazonas, Brazil

ScienciaScripts

SUMMARY

I dedicate this work to you,

To God, for his willpower and companionship;

To my mother, Lenise, and my brother Fabian, for their encouragement, patience and understanding;

To my daughter Natalie, for all her affection and love;

ACKNOWLEDGMENTS

To the Sao Leopoldo Mandic Dental Research Center, for providing the necessary structure for the master's course and the development of this work.

To Prof. Dr. Antonio Sergio Guimaraes, course coordinator, for his guidance and knowledge.

To the teachers, for their support over the months.

To all my colleagues on the course, especially my friend Marley, for their companionship, friendship and good memories.

To the Patients, for their simplicity and greatness in allowing us to learn.

SUMMARY

The aim of this study was to assess the knowledge of orthodontists and/or functional jaw orthopedists in Amazonas about temporomandibular dysfunction (TMD) and compare it with the results of similar studies. The sample consisted of 98 specialists out of a total of 137 registered with the CRO-AM, assessed using a questionnaire developed at the University of Washington (USA) and previously used in other studies in the United States, Korea and Brazil. The translated questionnaire consisted of 35 statements from four areas related to TMD: a) physiopathology, relating to the biomedical and biomechanical aspects of TMD (13 items); b) psychophysiology, referring to the interaction of physical and psychological factors in the etiology, diagnosis and treatment of TMD (9 items); c) chronic pain, relating to the cause, diagnosis and treatment of chronic conditions applied to TMD (9 items); and d) psychiatric disorders, about anxiety, depression or somatization, sometimes related to TMD (4 items). After collection and tabulation, the data was compared with the opinions of TMD experts on these items, using the Test of Equality of Two Proportions (p-value < 0.05). The results of the sample agreed with the experts on the items on psychiatric disorders, but differed from their opinion on the items on pathophysiology, psychophysiology and chronic pain. It was concluded that orthodontists and/or functional jaw orthopedists in Amazonas widely recognize the importance of psychiatric disorders and psychophysiological factors in the etiology and development of TMD; they were unaware of the use of medication in TMD; had an occlusionist view of TMD treatment, as there was a considerable difference between the opinion of orthodontists in Manaus and TMD experts on the pathophysiology of TMD and the diagnosis and treatment of chronic pain; the data found and discussed are similar to those found in studies carried out in Seattle, Kansas, Seoul and Brasilia.

Keywords: Temporomandibular dysfunction. TMD. Knowledge

1   INTRODUCTION

Temporomandibular dysfunction (TMD) is a collective term that covers a broad spectrum of clinical problems of the joints and muscles of the orofacial area (Carlsson et al., 2006).

Historically, McNeill (1997a) stated that the treatment of TMD began with the ancient Egyptians manipulating dislocated mandibles. The late 19th century revealed a more aggressive treatment of TMD, with surgeons repositioning or removing articular discs. In 1934, James Costen published that head, ear and jaw pain improved with a "bite lift", and with this began the occlusal treatment of TMD. Also, in the mid-20th century, many dentists became interested in joint popping and complex occlusal techniques to relieve the signs and symptoms of TMD. Although most, if not all, of Costen's and the clinicians' hypotheses were challenged by anatomists and physiologists, many dentists, and especially orthodontists, continued to accept the concept that structural disharmonies were the primary cause of TMD and therefore numerous irreversible procedures were performed (McNeill, 1997a).

Even today, there is a great deal of debate about the etiology of TMD, with the most widely accepted being an association of factors: predisposing factors, which increase the risk of TMD; initiating factors, which are responsible for its onset; and perpetuating factors, which interfere with healing or contribute to the maintenance and progression of the disease (Venâncio, Camparis, 2002).

According to Moana Filho (2005), TMD has often been related to orthodontic treatment, given the significant number of literature reviews and studies produced on the subject in recent years (Just et al., 1991; Casagrande, Rossato, 1998; Luther, 1998a; Luther, 1998b; McNamara Jr., 1997; Mao, Duan, 2001; Machado et al., 2010), including a meta-analysis (Kim et al., 2002). The only safe conclusion to be drawn from reading these articles is that this subject is permeated by controversy. Therefore, the dental profession is certainly divided as to how these dysfunctions should be conceptualized, diagnosed and treated.

Some studies have been carried out using questionnaires to clarify the knowledge and opinions of DSs and orthodontists, which have shown a difference between what specialists in the field know and what professionals practice in their offices (Le Resche et al., 1993; Glaros et al.,1994; Francesquini Jr. et al., 1999, Moana Filho, 2005, Tegelberg et al., 2001; Tegelberg et al., 2007; Ribeiro, 2009; Baharvand et al., 2010).

Thus, the aim of this study was to evaluate the opinions of orthodontists and/or functional jaw orthopedists on the concepts associated with TMD, professional conduct, types and characteristics of the treatments used, providing an overview of current information and action in this area, as well as comparing them with the results of similar studies carried out in the past in Brasilia, Kansas, Seoul, Seattle and Sweden. Based on this, we may or may not suggest a TMD education program for orthodontists in the state of Amazonas.

2   LITERATURE review

Just et al. (1991) used a questionnaire to assess the beliefs of various groups of dentists about the symptoms, causes and diagnosis of TMD, as well as the role of malocclusions and orthodontic treatment methods in the development of these disorders. To do this, the authors chose five specific groups to administer the questionnaire, based on their involvement in TMD or orthodontics. A total of 4,400 questionnaires were sent to members of the American Academy of General Practice Orthodontics (AAGPO), the American Equilibrium Society (AES), the American Academy of Craniomandibular Disorders (AACD), the American Association of Functional Orthodontists (AAFO) and the American Association of Orthodontics (AAO). Of which 1,402 (32 percent) were answered.

The survey included 75 questions on specific topics, such as the signs and symptoms of TMD and the contribution, to the treatment and development of TMD, of various malocclusions and types of orthodontic treatment, such as pre-molar extractions, Class II elastics, braces, and the use of various diagnostic aids for this dysfunction, among other questions.

They concluded that there was greater agreement on the importance of psychophysiological factors and the role they play in the development of TMD than in the 1973 study. However, the groups' opinions still conflicted, reflecting their educational and philosophical backgrounds. In addition, their opinions differed from the scientific literature of the time in several respects. Some of them are listed below:

Although scientific studies have not established any consistent relationships between malocclusions and the development of TMD, between two-thirds and three-quarters of respondents from all groups believed that all malocclusions can contribute to the development of TMD. Two-thirds of AAFO respondents believed that Class II Division 2 and deep bite were important factors in the development of TMD.

Three-quarters of AAO respondents did not believe that pre-molar extraction was related to the development of TMD, which agreed with the scientific literature, however, 80% of AAFO members and more than half of the members of the other three groups thought that pre-molar extraction contributed to the development of TMD.

Around 60% of AES, AAGPO and AACD respondents and 82% of AAFO members believed that it was possible or even likely that there would be a higher incidence of TMD in people who had been treated with conventional orthodontic therapy. 84% of AAO members found this relationship unlikely. Recent studies by many researchers have been unable to establish any link between orthodontic treatment and the development of TMD.

Although some studies have shown a poor prognosis for the treatment of TMJ clicks, and guidelines generally recommend avoiding the treatment of asymptomatic clicks, 35% to 49% of respondents from the AAFO, AES, AAGPO and AACD think that an asymptomatic click should be treated before orthodontics. However, 86% of AAO members responded that an asymptomatic click should not be treated before orthodontic treatment.

Transcranial radiographs of the TMJ have little diagnostic value, but 50% of AAFO, AES and AAGPO members believe that these radiographs should be used to diagnose TMD. In contrast, only 8% of AAO members gave a similar response.

Two-thirds of respondents from all groups believed that an asymptomatic click could be the precursor to more serious TMD problems, however, recent long-term studies have shown that this is generally untrue.

The authors concluded that although research has allowed for a better understanding of the cause, diagnosis and treatment of TMD, the large discrepancy between the scientific literature and the opinions presented in this study represent a general lack of knowledge about some of the research in the last 10 years in the area of temporomandibular disorders, although it should be pointed out that AAO members were more likely to have opinions that were supported by scientific evidence.

Le Resche et al. (1993) surveyed 386 dentists, including 181 clinicians and 212 specialists in orthodontics, oral medicine, oral and maxillofacial surgery, endodontics, periodontics and prosthodontics in Seattle, Washington State, USA, in order to obtain information on the causes, diagnosis and treatment of TMD.

They developed a questionnaire with statements taken from postgraduate courses in TMD, continuing education courses and articles published on the subject, which were evaluated by specialists and researchers, also called experts and recognized for working in multidisciplinary centers as well as developing scientific work on the subject. Each statement was answered using an 11-point sequential scale, between "0" and "10", where zero is "totally disagree" and 10 is "totally agree". An item was considered a "consensus" among the experts if it received 75% "agree" ("7" to "10" on the scale) or "disagree" ("0" to "3" on the scale) and less than 10% expressed the opposite opinion.

Only the statements with the highest levels of agreement among the experts were included in the questionnaire. The responses of the group of experts were used as a reference for assessing the knowledge of the dentists surveyed. This group was made up of 13 dentists who are members of the neuroscience group of the International Association for Dental Research (IADR) or the International Association for the Study of Pain (IASP), who publish extensively in the field and most of whom have extensive clinical and academic experience with TMD. Of these, seven were affiliated with multidisciplinary pain management programs at university centers. In addition, in the area of chronic pain and psychiatric disorders, 14 psychologists from multidisciplinary clinical centers for chronic pain served as references in these areas.

This methodology selected 35 statements from four areas related to TMD: a) physiopathology, concerning the biomedical and biomechanical aspects of TMD (thirteen items); b) psychophysiology, concerning the interaction of physical and psychological factors in the etiology, diagnosis and treatment of TMD (nine items); c) chronic pain, concerning the cause, diagnosis and treatment of chronic conditions applied to TMD (nine items) and; d) psychiatric disorders, concerning anxiety, depression or somatization, sometimes related to TMD (four items).

Regarding the pathophysiology of TMD, the specialists' opinions were significantly closer to those of the experts than those of the general practitioners. There was no significant difference in the opinion of the groups surveyed regarding the effectiveness of heat, cold and stretching therapies, the relationship between nocturnal bruxism and occlusal interferences, except for the effectiveness of repositioning plates. The section on occlusal treatments and theories as a cause of TMD had the lowest level of agreement between the experts and the groups surveyed.

In contrast to the area of pathophysiology, in the area of TMD psychophysiology there was no significant difference between the responses of specialists and general practitioners. The level of agreement was high between the groups surveyed and the experts. It was noted that the professionals interviewed saw stress control as an appropriate treatment.

In the area of chronic pain, the specialists agreed with the experts more than the general practitioners on the use of antidepressants in the management of TMD and on the inappropriate use of narcotics and surgery in cases of persistent pain. Both groups surveyed believed that patients with chronic pain should be advised to reduce professional and social activities. This opinion contrasted with the experts, who suggested the opposite, namely increasing these activities during the chronic phase of pain to avoid the development of disabling pain behavior.

Regarding psychiatric disorders, there was a high level of agreement between the dentists surveyed and the experts. However, the group of specialists was more biased than the general practitioners in agreeing with the experts who stated that depressive behavior was common in TMD patients, and that clinical depression occurred commonly in these patients.

The authors concluded that the role of psychophysiological factors in TMD was well known among Seattle dentists. However, there was still controversy about the pathophysiology of the problem. The differences in responses between experts and interviewees were based, according to the researchers, on an unfounded lack of knowledge or arguments on both sides on the subject, resulting in a confused opinion. Thus, it was realized that continuing education programs had not reached the group of clinical dentists and that research on TMD should be part of the clinicians' literature in order to improve their understanding of the subject. It was therefore suggested that further research be carried out to assess how dentists' personal characteristics and practices interfere with their knowledge and beliefs, which directly influence how and when they treat TMD.

Glass et al. (1993) conducted a survey of 10,000 members of the American Dental Association in order to identify the most commonly used treatments for the treatment of myofascial pain. A questionnaire was used in which the disease was defined, all treatments (including referral to other professionals) were listed, and an estimated percentage use for each treatment was requested. The results of 2544 questionnaires showed that the most commonly used treatments are: flat surface plates with canine guidance or group function, occlusal balancing, thermotherapy, muscle relaxation techniques, diet counseling and medication with anti-inflammatory (non-opioid) analgesics and muscle relaxants. The results also showed a considerable variation in the ways in which these treatments were carried out.

The following year, Glaros et al. (1994) published a survey of dentists in the Kansas metropolitan area, in the United States, on TMD and chronic pain, using the same questionnaire applied in Seattle. They selected 25% of clinical dentists, totaling 169, and 25% of specialists in the Kansas metropolitan area, excluding pediatric dentists and pathologists, totaling 34 professionals.

The questionnaire was sent by post between May and June 1991 and, unlike the survey carried out in Seattle, no financial incentive was offered to the participants. A total of 104 questionnaires were sent to clinical dentists and 21 to specialists. In a preliminary analysis, there was no significant difference in the responses of the two groups. Therefore, all the answers were combined and compared to the opinion of the same experts from the Seattle study. Fisher's exact test was also used in the statistics to compare the data with a 1% margin of error.

The data collected suggested that the pathophysiology and psychiatric disorders in the etiology of TMD were widely known by DCs. However, there was considerable discrepancy in the opinions of dentists and experts on pathophysiology and chronic pain related to TMD. The results obtained partially replicated the research carried out in Seattle. The authors suggested continuing education and the review of scientific articles to reduce the gap between advances in the field and daily practice. These two methods of updating knowledge, in the authors' opinion, could still prevent the diagnosis and adoption of therapies with no scientific basis.

In 1997, McNamara Jr. carried out a literature review of 90 publications linking orthodontic treatment with TMD, since several clinical studies had been conducted in the 1980s to investigate this association. This interest in orthodontics and TMD arose following several lawsuits in the United States, alleging that orthodontic treatment was the cause of TMD in these patients. This litigious climate resulted in a greater understanding of the need for risk management, as well as for conducting clinical studies. The research findings revealed that: (1) signs and symptoms of TMD can occur in healthy people; (2) signs and symptoms of TMD increase with age, especially during adolescence until menopause, so TMD that originates during orthodontic treatment cannot be related to the treatment, (3) in general, orthodontic treatment performed during adolescence does not increase or decrease the likelihood of developing TMD later in life, and (4) tooth extraction as part of an orthodontic treatment plan does not increase the risk of TMD, (5) there is no increased risk of TMD associated with any type of orthodontic mechanics; (6) although a stable occlusion is the goal of good orthodontic treatment, not achieving it does not result in signs and symptoms of TMD; and (7) so far, there is little evidence that orthodontic treatment prevents TMD, although the role of correcting unilateral posterior crossbite in children may merit further investigation.

McNeill, still in 1997a, wrote that TMD control was carried out on the basis of belief systems and statements according to the clinician's favorite theory. The common assumption was that good health depended on specific morphological criteria. It was believed that an abnormal variation in interocclusal, interarch or intra-articular relationship predisposed the tissues of the masticatory system to dysfunction or disease. However, preconceived ideals based on morphology rather than function may have little or no relation to masticatory health. A morphological variation with no evidence of pathological tissue may actually be a developmental adaptation, by whatever combination of intrinsic and extrinsic factors that results in functional balance being the most physiological relationship for that particular individual. As a result of these morphological beliefs, treatment for TMD has often in the past been carried out using a mechanical restorative approach, rather than a global multidisciplinary approach.

In the same year, McNeill (1997b) wrote about the controversy in the field of TMD epidemiology, etiology, diagnosis and treatment. He defined different types of joint and muscle TMD and TMD treatments, from occlusal, orthodontic, physiotherapeutic to drug and surgical, found in the literature. From this literature review, it was concluded that little is known about the natural course of TMD, and as most types of treatment are reported to be equally effective, a conservative, non-invasive treatment program should be endorsed. The emphasis should be on a multidisciplinary treatment model of health professionals similar to those used for other musculoskeletal disorders that involve the patient in the physical and behavioral management of their problem.

Following the trend of the decade, Luther (1998a) also carried out a literature review relating orthodontic treatment to TMD, and another relating functional occlusion and malocclusion to TMD (Luther, 1998b). In the first, after reading 51 articles on the subject, the author concluded that although the "perfect" study relating orthodontics to TMD had not yet been carried out, there was a strong trend suggesting that orthodontic treatment neither causes nor prevents TMD. Even though some studies have claimed that orthodontic treatment cures TMD, they are not enough to direct TMD treatment towards orthodontics, because they were case reports which, on their own, cannot be considered evidence. In part 2 of the article, after reviewing 51 other articles, he concluded that just like orthodontic treatment, malocclusion does not cause TMD and correcting it does not cure it.

The Brazilian Francesquini Jr et al. (1999) applied a questionnaire with structured, semi-structured and open questions, divided into professional identification and technical information, to four groups, one of dentists and three of academics. Group I was made up of students from the 4th period of their dental degree at FOP/UNICAMP, Group II, students from the 6th period and Group III, from the 8th period of the same institution. Finally, group IV was made up of professionals from the cities of Aguas de São Pedro, Capivari, Charqueada, Elias Fausto, Mombuca, Rafard, Rio das Pedras, Saltinho, Santa Maria da Serra, São Pedro and Piracicaba. The authors concluded that the majority of academics and professionals in the groups had insufficient knowledge of the anatomy and physiology of the TMJ and attached structures, as well as the pathologies that affect it. With regard to complementary exams, the majority were unable to list the exams needed to establish a differential diagnosis. Less than 75% of the population in the groups use a standardized sequence of exams to establish TMD and the vast majority of those interviewed feel the need for a continuing education program in the area of diagnosis and treatment. Finally, 75% consider themselves unfit to diagnose and treat TMD.

In 1999, Forsell et al. carried out a systematic review of the literature from 1966 to 1999 entitled "Occlusal treatments in temporomandibular disorders: a qualitative systematic review of randomized clinical trials", in which they selected 18 studies by their inclusion criteria, 14 of which concerned occlusal plates and 4 occlusal adjustments. According to them, they were unable to conclude anything very significant since most of the studies had flaws such as small sample size, inadequate patient and/or operator blinding, insufficient follow-up and a wide variety of outcome measures. The authors suggest that occlusal plate therapy may be beneficial for the treatment of TMD and can conclude nothing about occlusal adjustment, and recommend that more controlled studies be carried out in order to draw better conclusions.

Lee et al. (2000) applied the same Seattle questionnaire that was mentioned at the beginning of this review to dentists in Seoul. They assessed the knowledge of Korean dentists in the area of TMD diagnosis and treatment, with the aim of duplicating the Seattle study as closely as possible.

The Washington University questionnaire, after translation into Korean and revision with pilot testing, was mailed to 1000 dentists under the age of 60 in the city of Seoul. The sample was randomly selected from the list of licensed dentists in the city. Data collection took place during 1996 and, even after three contacts by letter or telephone, there were only 76 respondents.

The majority of respondents were male, in private practice, there were few specialists and they rarely treated TMD. These dentists usually referred TMD patients to pain clinics located in universities. According to the authors, there was no difference in the responses of the specialists and general practitioners surveyed. Therefore, the responses of these groups were combined and compared to the opinion of the experts.

The authors concluded by stating that the data obtained suggested that dentists in Seoul tended to agree with the experts on the role of psychiatric disorders in the etiology and psychophysiology of TMD. However, there was considerable divergence in the fields of TMD pathophysiology and the diagnosis and treatment of chronic pain situations. Further research was suggested into how the knowledge of dentists in Seoul interfered with the choice of when and how to treat TMD. Another suggestion was to reduce the gap between scientific advances in the field of TMD and private practice by using continuing education guided by scientific articles. It was also pointed out that these results were similar to those found in Seattle and Kansas, but should not be extrapolated to other populations.

In 2001, in order to carry out a qualitative and quantitative analysis of the use of a diagnostic tool,

Manfredi et al. (2001) applied the "Questionnaire for Screening for Orofacial Pain and TMD", recommended by the American Academy of Orofacial Pain, which had not yet been tested in Brazil at that time. The target population was patients with complaints of non-tooth pain in the orofacial region, headache, otalgia and/or TMJ who came to the medical and dental outpatient clinic at Unicamp. The questionnaire, made up of 10 yes/no questions, was administered to 46 patients (40 women and 6 men) followed by a specific clinical examination for the diagnosis of TMD. The examination consisted of anamnesis, palpation of muscles and TMJ, as well as assessment of dental trauma, orthodontic treatment and maximum mouth opening.

They observed that the questionnaire had a sensitivity of 85.37% and a specificity of 80% for patients with muscle alterations in the orofacial region. Low sensitivity and specificity were also found for intra-articular disorders. The authors concluded that the use of the questionnaire was useful and feasible in the pre-screening of TMD sufferers, especially muscle alterations, however, the questionnaire should not be used as the only resource for diagnosis. Furthermore, the need for multidisciplinary assessment of patients with headaches was essential.

In the same year, Mao & Duan (2001) evaluated the relationship between orthodontic treatment and temporomandibular disorders among Chinese orthodontists. They used a 10-question questionnaire and administered it to 25 orthodontists from public hospitals in Xian, China.

The questionnaire included questions such as: Do you ask patients if they have any signs and symptoms of TMD before starting orthodontic treatment? Do you palpate the masticatory muscles, TMJ and check mandibular position in your patients before orthodontic treatment? Whether before, during or after orthodontic treatment the patients had signs of pain, discomfort or sensations of noise or clicking in the TMJ or facial area; difficulties or changes in jaw movements? Does orthodontic treatment have an effect on: muscles of mastication; TMJ; mandibular position (condylar position)? Can orthodontic treatment lead to a higher incidence of TMD? Does orthodontic treatment prevent TMD?

The results showed that 84% of orthodontists frequently asked their patients about the signs and symptoms of TMD before orthodontic treatment and 92% reported examining the TMJ region. 76% of orthodontists believe that orthodontic treatment can eventually lead to a higher incidence of TMD, while 84% stated that orthodontic treatment can prevent TMD. The respondents answered that orthodontic treatment, patient age, and occlusal interferences are risk factors that lead to an increased incidence of TMD.

Also in 2001, Tegelberg et al. (2001) published a survey in Sweden on dentists' attitudes, routine and experience with TMD in children and adolescents. A questionnaire, applied in three municipalities in Sweden: Ostergotland, Vastmanland, and Gothenburg, was sent to 286 public service dentists.

The questionnaire contained 13 questions in the following areas: A) demographic information such as gender, the number of years in the profession, the number of patients being treated in the 0-19 age group, and the number of children and adolescents, with TMD, treated during 1998. B) Quality assurance indicated whether the professional uses a health declaration containing questions about orofacial pain and headache in TMD, whether they regularly record the history of pain and mouth opening in the patients' records, and whether they participate in continuing education in TMD. The questions were answered with yes or no. C) Clinical experience and treatment, which assessed diagnostic ability, therapeutic decisions, treatment results and a report on the frequency of patients undergoing treatment. These questions were answered on a 3-point scale; 0 = lack of routine / unable, 1 = limited routine / unsure, 2 = good routine / confident. Finally, at this stage, the frequency of seven decisions on how to proceed with a patient were ranked in descending order (information and talk therapy, occlusal balance, occlusal plate, jaw exercise, pharmacological interventions, referrals to TMD specialists, and referrals to physiotherapists). D) The need for specialized resources for a consultation in their own clinic, either to refer to a specialized clinic, for a telephone consultation, for the possibility of auscultation, or the need for continuing education. The questions were answered with yes or no. E) Attitude: The statement: "The treatment of children and adolescents with pain is ... " should be answered with two of the following adjectives: interesting, educational, rewarding, worthwhile, stressful, difficult, frustrating, unpleasant, difficult, demanding. The dentists had to choose two of the alternatives to finish the sentence. Five of the adjectives were considered positive and 5 negative. The dentist's attitude was considered positive if both adjectives were positive, neutral if one was positive and one negative, and negative if both were negative.

Eighty-seven percent (250) of the dentists answered the questionnaire. Dentists in the three municipalities reported good routine and safety in occlusal plate treatments (74% - 81%), occlusal balancing (28% - 55%), mandibular exercises (25% - 29%), and medication treatments (3% - 55%). Good experience with diagnosis and therapeutic decision-making was reported by 25% - 50% of dentists. A larger proportion of the dentists in Vastmanland had attended TMD courses compared to the other two municipalities. Recordings of verbal and/or written case histories with questions about facial pain and tension-type headache (1% - 39%) and measurements of mouth openings were performed more frequently in the three municipalities (0% - 5%). 55% of dentists had a positive attitude towards caring for children and adolescents with TMD. The great need for specialized resources with the possibility of sending referrals or consulting was reported by 98% - 100% of respondents, to participate in continuing education by 97% - 98%, and to perform auscultation by 61% - 82%.

In conclusion, many of the dentists did not have routines for making diagnoses, deciding on therapy, and judging treatment results. Good routines were reported only in occlusal plate therapy. Most dentists had a positive attitude towards caring for children and adolescents with TMD-related symptoms. Most dentists reported a great need for specialists in the field.

Wright & Sluka (2001) studied the evidence for each of the types of non-drug therapy indicated for the treatment of musculoskeletal pain. The most common types of therapy could be divided into: a) electrotherapy, such as transcutaneous electrical nerve stimulation (TENS); b) acupuncture; c) thermal therapies, such as ultrasound and moist heat; d) manual therapies, such as manipulation or massage and; e) exercise. Within each of these broad categories, there was a significant variation in treatment parameters, taking into account reports of clinical effectiveness and scientific studies evaluating the potential therapeutic effects of each treatment modality.

The authors found evidence to suggest that there could be potential therapeutic effects, although there were few quality randomized clinical trials to support the therapeutic effectiveness of various types of treatment. In other words, although there was a good scientific basis, the effectiveness could not be translated into clear evidence for the clinical environment. In addition, research was needed into how each of these therapies acted on the endogenous pain control mechanism.

Finally, they concluded that a prudent combination of treatment modalities could produce a significant therapeutic effect and that there was still a clear need for more research in this area.

Venâncio & Camparis (2002) set out to find out the percentage of professionals who treated TMD, as well as the types and characteristics of the treatments used and to assess their opinion on the etiology of TMD. A total of 150 12-question questionnaires were sent to DCs and specialists in the city of Ribeirao Preto, located in the state of Sao Paulo. Specialists who worked only in endodontics and pediatric dentistry were excluded from the sample. A total of 100 questionnaires were used, as some were not returned or were returned incomplete.

The authors reported that most of the professionals interviewed had already received patients with painful symptoms in the region of the masticatory muscles and TMJ, and had been referred by other health professionals. It was found that controversy persisted over the etiology and treatment of TMD, and that a significant proportion of those interviewed used irreversible treatments such as occlusal adjustment, although they believed in conservative and multidisciplinary treatments for TMD.

They then concluded that TMD diagnosis and treatment concepts did not yet have the desired scientific support and that it was up to the dentist to be up-to-date and seek individual diagnosis for their patients.

Due to a lack of knowledge about the causes of TMD, Kim et al. (2002) in a meta-analysis on orthodontics and TMD found that the articles had methodological flaws and lacked a widely accepted classification scheme. For this reason, perhaps, they were unable to draw definitive conclusions. The data from this meta-analysis does not indicate that traditional orthodontic treatment increases the prevalence of TMD.

In 2004, Forssell & Kalso wrote with the aim of elucidating and discussing the application of evidence-based medicine (EBM) in the treatment of TMD with very controversial methods, such as occlusal treatments. EBM meant the systematic, explicit and prudent use of the best evidence in patient care. This view would be particularly interesting in TMD, as it is a field of much debate and controversy. Furthermore, it was still very common to cite a lack of scientific evidence.

The authors explained that the most reliable source of scientific evidence came from high-quality systematic reviews and randomized controlled trials (RCTs). The systematic review of occlusal therapies (splints, plates and occlusal adjustment) up to January 2003 showed 16 RCTs of occlusal plates and four of occlusal adjustment. However, the quality of these studies was insufficient, but had improved in recent years. The problems with these studies were their methodology, inadequate execution and short-term follow-up, among others. As a result, the authors realized, for example, that studies with occlusal plates yielded erroneous results.

It was concluded that even in the most studied area - stabilizing plates for myofascial pain, the results did not justify definitive conclusions about the effectiveness of occlusal plates. The clinical effectiveness of the relief obtained also seemed modest when compared to common pain treatment methods. None of the studies on occlusal adjustment led to proven support for using such a treatment method.

The authors also described EBM as the integration of individual clinical expertise with the best available evidence, moderated by the patient's preferences and circumstances, with the focus being on improving patient care.

In 2005, Parashos et al. wrote an article with the aim of describing the response rate and non-response trends of a survey using questionnaires for dentists, and also to make recommendations for future research using questionnaires in dentistry. They describe a survey that collected data using a questionnaire sent by post. Three mailings of the questionnaire, telephone contact, postage-paid return envelopes and personalized correspondence were used as strategies to increase the respondent rate.

According to the authors, there were several methods to compensate for the low return rate and increase responses without interfering with the quality of the surveys. They suggested using various techniques associated with this objective, including personalized correspondence, postal follow-up, telephone contact, financial and material incentives. The researchers realized that a single contact was probably sufficient for collecting survey data and that multiple attempts to increase the response rate were recommended. However, the data obtained indicated that there would be little difference in the results if the remaining non-respondents cooperated.

It was also asked whether behavioral factors could have influenced data collection, such as: the first respondents were probably more interested in the topic of the survey or were the most active professionals in the dental community.

Also in 2005, Moana Filho, in Brazil, evaluated the attitudes and beliefs of orthodontists regarding temporomandibular dysfunction and orofacial pain through a questionnaire sent by e-mail to orthodontists registered with the Brazilian Association of Orthodontics (ABOR), consisting of nine questions regarding demographic information and academic training; Continuing education in

TMD/OFD; Knowledge of the occurrence of TMD/OFD; Clinical experience and treatment of TMD/OFD in their patients; Need for specialists in the area of TMD/OFD in the participant's region; Beliefs about the relationship between orthodontic treatment and TMD/OFD.

Most of the participants reported having obtained basic or no knowledge of TMD/OFD during their post-graduate orthodontic course; most of the interviewees did not feel confident about diagnosing, making therapeutic decisions and evaluating the results of TMD/OFD treatment; the most commonly used therapy was occlusal plates among the participants; the vast majority of interviewees believe that orthodontic treatment does not lead to a higher incidence of TMD/OFD, but they do believe that it can be a form of prevention and treatment of these dysfunctions; 52.4% of interviewees believe that there is a need for a TMD/OFD specialist in their region, where patient referral and the promotion of continuing education in TMD/OFD would be the most frequent reasons for this need.

Mohl & Ohrbach (2006) discussed the dilemma between scientific knowledge and clinical management of TMD. The authors evaluated the issue by looking at five questions: a) what was scientific evidence and how was it transmitted? b) what important evidence was missing in the field of TMD? c) which clinical concepts should be confronted by scientific evidence? d) why was there still adherence to concepts that apparently confront scientific evidence? and; e) how did the clinician promote treatment to patients based on the uncertain while maintaining scientific integrity?

It was concluded that there was no justifiable reason for the dilemma between scientific evidence and clinical need, as long as: a) researchers used appropriate research protocols and presented the results in scientific journals; and b) dentists were familiar with the requirements of scientific evidence and interpreted this evidence and its clinical implications, applying it to the treatment of TMD patients.

In the same year, Medlicott & Harris (2006) carried out a systematic review of several studies that analyzed the effectiveness of various physiotherapy interventions for temporomandibular dysfunction. The search was restricted to publications in English from 1966 to January 2005 and based on four criteria: (1) patients were diagnosed by the first axis of the RDC/TMD (Research Diagnostic Criteria for Temporomandibular Disorders) (2), the intervention carried out was within physiotherapy practice, (3) an experimental design was used, and (4) the outcome was the treatment of one or more of the main symptoms presented. Of the 108 articles with an experimental model, most included drug and surgical treatment, so they were excluded, leaving only thirty studies. Four randomly selected articles were independently classified by two evaluators (100% agreement for levels of evidence and 73.5% for methodological rigor).

The following recommendations emerged from the 30 studies: (1) active exercises and manual therapies may be effective, (2) postural training may be used in combination with other interventions, (3) laser therapy may be more effective than other electrotherapy modalities, (4) programs involving relaxation techniques and biofeedback, electromyography, and proprioceptive reeducation may be more effective than placebo treatment or occlusal plates, and (5) combinations of active exercises, manual therapy, postural correction, and relaxation techniques may be effective.

In 2007, Tegelberg et al. published a study carried out with the collaboration of three counties in Sweden: Ostergotland, Vastmanland and Gothenburg. A questionnaire was sent randomly to 100 dentists in each of these cities and to all 87 in Vastmanland so that the samples were similar in size. All three groups worked in the Public Dental Service with children and adolescents. The mail survey was also sent to 19 TMD specialists who had documented research activities and were members of the Swedish Academy of Temporomandibular Disorders. They formed the reference group of TMD specialists.

The questionnaire contained 37 statements about etiology, diagnosis, classification, chronic pain, pain behavior, treatment and prognosis. Each statement was judged on a 0-10 point scale with the terminal definitions agree or disagree. This questionnaire was based on that of the University of Washington in Seattle (Le Resche et al., 1993), with some modifications to direct the research towards dentists' knowledge of temporomandibular disorders in children and adolescents.

The overall response rate to the questionnaire was 87%. In 28 of the 37 statements, the TMD specialists approved a consensus, i.e. more than 75% of the specialists had the same opinion on the statement. TMD specialists differed most in their opinion in the field of TMD diagnosis and classification. In 65% of the statements, the differences in knowledge between DCs and TMD specialists were not significant. The greatest number of significant differences between the groups was found in the area of TMD treatment and prognosis. Most of these statements were related to morphological factors.

They concluded that there is a high degree of consensus in TMD knowledge among TMD specialists and a high degree of agreement in knowledge among clinicians and TMD specialists. In some areas, however, TMD specialists have yet to reach a consensus that is based on evidence-based knowledge of TMD in children and adolescents and that can be used in undergraduate teaching. Therefore, it is important to develop and strengthen undergraduate dental education in TMD/ODD.

Ribeiro (2009) replicated the study by Le Resche et al. (1993) for DCs in Brasilia - DF. Their aim was to assess the knowledge of dentists in Brasilia about temporomandibular dysfunction and compare it with the results of similar studies. The sample consisted of 138 dentists, the majority of whom were female (58%), with a mean age of 31.2 years, assessed using a questionnaire developed at the University of Washington (USA) and previously used in other studies in the United States and Korea. The questionnaire, which was translated and validated by a pilot test, consisted of the same 35 statements as the study by Le Resche et al. (1993).

After collection and tabulation, the data was compared with the opinions of TMD experts. The sample tended to agree with the experts on psychophysiology and psychiatric disorders, but tended to differ from their opinion on pathophysiology and chronic pain. It was concluded that dentists in Brasilia widely recognize the importance of psychiatric disorders and psychophysiological factors in the etiology and development of TMD. However, there was still controversy about the pathophysiology of TMD and the diagnosis and treatment of chronic pain. Similar results were found in samples of dentists from the cities of Seattle, Kansas and Seoul.

Michelotti & Iodice (2010) carried out a literature review of 139 articles on the role of orthodontics in temporomandibular disorders. They concluded that because TMD is a multifactorial pathology, it was difficult to demonstrate a direct relationship between one of the possible causes, such as occlusion. They commented that there were so many variables in the studies that they did not have adequate diagnostic tools to establish a clear correlation or to know when and how a bad occlusion could unbalance the stomatognathic system. It is important to rule out other causes of facial pain before investigating teeth as a potential etiological factor.

When the treatment protocol included dental intervention, this should be done to resolve the patient's discomfort and achieve a stable occlusion. It shows the importance of bearing in mind that dysfunctional patients have a lower capacity to adapt to occlusal changes, because they seem to be more vigilant in their occlusion and are easily disturbed by occlusal instability. Therefore, orthodontic treatment must be carried out in accordance with the rules that allow a stable occlusion to be achieved.

He commented that various therapeutic protocols have been suggested for TMD. As a consequence of the multifactorial etiology, a non-invasive multidisciplinary therapy is generally suggested, with reversible treatments for TMD. Therefore, treatments must address not only the physical diagnosis, but also the psychological and psychosocial suffering of the dysfunction found in patients affected by chronic pain conditions. In fact, the severity of the case and chronicity represent critical factors in the decision-making process. When severe pain is present, occlusal treatments (such as orthodontics and prosthodontics) should be postponed until symptoms improve. There is a current consensus that treatment strategies should be reversible. This therapeutic approach is supported by evidence showing that no one treatment modality has been proven to be better than another. Long-term follow-up of TMD patients shows that 75-85% of patients with chronic pain are cured or significantly improved regardless of the treatment modality used.

When it comes to TMJ dysfunction, the goals of treatment should be to reduce pain and improve function. Reversible therapies commonly used for TMJ dysfunction include physiotherapy (to improve movement and function), pharmacotherapy (anti-inflammatories, antidepressants, etc.), occlusal therapy (occlusal appliances) and psychological therapy (cognitive-behavioral therapy). These modalities can be offered together or as a single strategy. Intra-oral appliances, such as occlusal stabilization plates, have been the main treatment for mandibular dysfunction for many decades and will continue to be a common treatment modality. Various hypotheses have been suggested to explain their action, but scientific validation is still lacking. Therefore, it is difficult to establish the effectiveness of plates in the treatment of TMD. Occlusal therapy should only be considered to resolve the TMD patient's discomfort.

Machado et al. (2010) carried out a systematic review of the literature on orthodontics as a risk factor for TMD. The search was carried out in the following databases: Medline, Cochrane, Embase,

Pubmed, Lilacs and BBO, between 1966 and 2009, focusing on randomized clinical trials, prospective and non-randomized longitudinal studies, systematic reviews and meta-analysis. After applying the inclusion criteria, 18 articles were selected, 12 of which were non-randomized prospective longitudinal studies, four systematic reviews, one randomized clinical trial and one meta-analysis, which assessed the relationship between orthodontic treatment and TMD. As expected, according to the literature, they concluded that orthodontic treatment cannot be considered a factor contributing to the development of temporomandibular disorders.

Baharvand et al. (2010) published a study in which a questionnaire containing 29 questions on the etiology, signs and symptoms, diagnosis and treatment of TMD was given to 200 randomly selected DCs and 11 TMD specialists, who were chosen from the academic staff of the Shaheed Beheshti University of Medical Sciences in Tehran, Iran. Considering the fact that they are more involved in the treatment of TMD patients than other dentists, their answers were taken as standard for comparison with other participants.

The questionnaire, which was taken from *J.P. Okeson*'s *Management of Temporomandibular Disorders and Occlusion, 5th ed. St Louis: Mosby; 2003*, was made up of three sections: knowledge, attitude and practice. The knowledge section consisted of 18 questions with answers (agree, disagree, indifferent), and a multiple choice question covering four signal domains, such as etiology, symptoms, diagnosis and treatment. The section on attitude consisted of five multiple-choice questions and yes/no questions in a clinical case presentation form, and the part on practice contained 5 multiple-choice questions on the respondents' opinion of accepting TMD patients, as well as acquiring sufficient knowledge about TMD and each practitioner's approach to this issue.

A response rate of 97% was achieved among the participants (average age: 39 ± 8.2 years old, average years in practice: 11.5 ± 7.4). The average TMD knowledge score was found to be 10.85 ± 2.54 (out of a total of 23). TMD specialists were significantly more experienced than dentists. With regard to attitude, there was a significant difference between the various age groups, and with increasing age and years of practice, the attitude towards TMD weakened. However, no significant difference was recorded between the attitude of dentists and TMD specialists towards TMD. There was a positive correlation between the subjects' knowledge and attitude. Thus, according to the results, the level of knowledge and attitude of Teera's general dentists about TMD is not desirable. Most of them are not willing to accept and treat TMD patients.

Grossman & Grossman (2011) reviewed the different surgical techniques used in TMD, as well as their indications. They observed that studies over the last few years have tried to standardize the different surgical techniques in order to define when and how to use them. They first opted for less invasive techniques such as assisted mandibular manipulation with increased hydrostatic pressure, arthrocentesis to more complex procedures such as arthroscopy and open TMJ surgery. They concluded that the choice of treatment for TMD depends much more on the experience and handling of the professional than on scientifically controlled studies and that the therapeutic success applied to the TMJ depends fundamentally on a global treatment plan that involves both conservative, clinical therapies and surgery itself. Surgery performed in isolation is unlikely to provide therapeutic success. Each procedure should have its own indication, based on well-defined criteria. However, to date, there is a lack of longitudinal studies and randomized clinical trials that can compare the therapeutic effectiveness of each surgical modality.

3   PROPOSAL

The proposal is to evaluate, by means of a questionnaire, the knowledge of orthodontists and/or functional jaw orthopedists in Amazonas about the area of TMD, by answering the following question:

What knowledge do orthodontists and/or functional jaw orthopedists in Amazonas have of the following areas related to TMD?

a)   Pathophysiology

b)   Psychophysiology

c)   Chronic pain

d)   Psychiatric disorders

4 MATERIAL AND METHOD

4.1 Clearance by the Ethics and Research Committee

The research project for this study was submitted to the Postgraduate Department of the CPO - Sao Leopoldo Mandic, and approved by the Research Ethics Committee, established at this University, at a meeting held on 04/04/2011, under protocol no. 20110032, in accordance with Resolution 196/1996 of the National Health Council - Ministry of Health (Annex A).

4.2 Sampling

The sample consisted of 98 orthodontists and/or functional jaw orthopedists. It was obtained from private practices and clinics. Almost all orthodontists and/or orthopedists in Manaus - AM (N=137) had access to the questionnaire, but the sample size corresponded to the number of questionnaires answered, which were returned to the researcher.

4.2.1 Inclusion Criteria

a)   registered with the Regional Council of Dentistry of Amazonas (CRO-AM) in the specialty of Orthodontics or Orthodontics and Functional Jaw Orthopedics or Functional Jaw Orthopedics;

b)   who practiced their profession in the state of Amazonas;

c)   who agreed to take part in the study by signing the informed consent form (Appendix B).

4.3 Questionnaire

The questionnaire used was the same one developed at the University of Washington in 1993, applied in the city of Seattle, translated and validated in the work of Ribeiro, 2009 (Appendix C).

Le Resche et al. (1993) developed a questionnaire with statements taken from TMD postgraduate courses, continuing education courses and articles published on the subject, which were evaluated by specialists and researchers, also known as experts, and recognized for working in multidisciplinary centers and for developing scientific work on the subject. Each statement was answered using an 11-point sequential scale, between "0" and "10", where zero is "totally disagree" and 10 is "totally agree". An item was considered a "consensus" among the experts if it received 75% "agree" ("7" to "10" on the scale) or "disagree" ("0" to "3" on the scale) and less than 10% expressed the opposite opinion.

The questionnaire only included the statements that were a consensus because they had the highest levels of agreement among the experts. The responses of the group of experts were used as a reference for assessing the knowledge of the orthodontists surveyed. This group was made up of 13 dentists who are members of the neuroscience group of the International Association for Dental Research (IADR) or the International Association for the Study of Pain (IASP), who publish extensively in the field and most of whom have extensive clinical and academic experience with TMD. Of these, seven were affiliated with multidisciplinary pain management programs at university centers. In addition, in the section on chronic pain and psychiatric disorders, 14 psychologists from multidisciplinary clinical centers for chronic pain served as references.

This methodology selected 35 statements from four areas related to TMD: a) physiopathology, concerning the biomedical and biomechanical aspects of TMD (thirteen items); b) psychophysiology, concerning the interaction of physical and psychological factors in the etiology, diagnosis and treatment of TMD (nine items); c) chronic pain, concerning the cause, diagnosis and treatment of chronic conditions applied to TMD (nine items) and; d) psychiatric disorders, concerning anxiety, depression or somatization, sometimes related to TMD (four items).

Each questionnaire was accompanied by an ICF (Annex B) for information and authorization to use the data collected, in which the objective of the work and the guarantee of confidentiality of personal and professional data were explained to each participant.

The first part of the questionnaire consisted of a brief explanation of how to answer the items. The numbered scale accompanying each statement in the questionnaire (Appendix C) was explained. The respondent had to mark with an "X" a single value, according to their knowledge or opinion. The participant was also asked to fill in all the fields and answer all the questions.

The second area was used to collect the respondents' personal academic data, such as: year of graduation, specialties completed and the respective year of completion, age and gender. To form the sample, the item "Do you provide care in Amazonas?" was also included in this section, followed by the alternatives "yes" and "no".

In line with the original work, the items were grouped into four areas relating to TMD, namely: pathophysiology, consisting of 13 items; psychophysiology, nine items; chronic pain, nine items and, finally, psychiatric disorders, only four items. Each item was given a sequential Arabic number, starting with "1", within each group.

Below are the items that made up the questionnaire.

4.3.1 Pathophysiology

a)   interference on the non-working side (balance) is commonly related to TMD;

b)   balancing occlusion is an early treatment for TMD;

c)   orthodontic treatment can prevent the onset of TMD;

d)   Surgical arthroscopy is almost completely effective in repositioning the disc in cases of internal joint disruption;

e)   Orthodontics is the best treatment for TMD in patients with skeletal malocclusion;

f)   TMD caused by trauma is much more difficult to treat and has a much worse prognosis than other types of TMD;

g)   Transcranial radiography is the most accurate method of visualizing the TMJ;

h)   the presence of joint changes on CT scans together with crepitus in the joints indicates the need for treatment;

i)   the position of the condyle in the fossa seen on a CT scan is an accurate indicator of joint disruption;

j)   lower repositioning plates are more effective than upper plates;

k)   nocturnal bruxism is caused by occlusal interference;

l)   Cold and/or heat followed by passive muscle stretching are good initial treatments for TMD;

m)   all individuals with TMJ clicks need treatment.

4.3.2 Psychophysiology

a)   the mechanisms of acute and chronic pain are the same;

b)   "biofeedback may be useless in the treatment of TMD;

c)   parafunctional habits are often important in the development of TMD;

d)   patients who grind and/or clench their teeth do so during the day or at night, never both;

e)   stress management is indicated for many TMD patients;

f)   stress is the main factor in the development of TMD;

g)   tension and stress increase chewing muscle activity in susceptible patients;

h)   Progressive muscle relaxation is not an effective treatment for TMD;

i)   Information on the daily pattern of TMD symptoms can be useful in identifying contributing factors.

4.3.3 Chronic pain

a)   patients with chronic TMD should be advised to rest and limit professional and social activities when in pain;

b)   narcotics (as "necessaries" for pain) are the treatment of choice when TMD pain is severe;

c)   antidepressants are never indicated in the management of TMD;

d)   an extensive history of failed treatments for TMD is a common indication for surgery;

e)   Chronic pain is a behavioral problem as well as a physical one;

f)   although some TMD patients have psychological problems, these problems are usually not related to pain;

g)   difficulty sleeping is a common finding in chronic pain;

h)   some patients use pain as an excuse to avoid unpleasant tasks;

i)   Behavior modification treatment is indicated for patients with chronic painful TMD.

4.3.4 Psychiatric disorders

a)   Clinical depression is rare in patients with chronic TMD;

b)   depressive behavior is common in TMD patients;

c)   Anxiety disorders are more common in TMD patients than in the general population;

d)   depression can be an important etiological factor in chronic pain.

4.4 Method

The printed questionnaires, accompanied by the respective ICF on a separate sheet, were distributed to private practices and clinics in the city of Manaus, Amazonas.

During data collection, which took place between January 2012 and February 2013, the author visited several practices in person, where he briefly explained the objectives and importance of the work to the specialists. The aim was to reduce the rate of non-responders. In addition, he made telephone contacts one week and two weeks after the questionnaire was delivered to collect it.

4.5 Methodologies

4.5.1 Statistics

The data was tabulated and the Test of Equality of Two Proportions was applied, a parametric test which compares whether the proportion of responses to two given variables and/or their levels are statistically significant. A significance level of 0.05 (α = 5%) was adopted, with descriptive levels (p) below this value being considered significant

4.5.2 Bibliography

The bibliographic *survey* was carried out in the Pubmed and Medline databases, using the keywords: *temporomandibular disorder, TMD, survey, knowledge, dentist, orthodontics*. Articles dealing with the knowledge of DCs and orthodontists about TMD were included in this study. Other studies cited in the bibliographical references of the selected articles were also added. However, papers were excluded if, although they included keywords, they did not have abstracts that correlated with the topic studied.

5   RESULTS

In the bibliographic review, 789 articles were found in Pubmed and 457 in Medline, and 1,215 were excluded. Articles whose abstracts were not compatible with the title and with this research, repeated articles, as well as those published in non-English were excluded. Papers from before 1990 were excluded. The total number of articles used was 31.

During the data collection period, the average age declared by the respondents (Graph 1) was 37.9 years with a standard deviation of 8.7 years. The youngest respondent was 25 years old and the oldest was 64 years old. Three respondents did not answer this item. The time since graduation (Graph 2) averaged 15.4 years with a standard deviation of 9.2 years, with a minimum of 4 and a maximum of 41 years. This item was answered by 91 of the 98 interviewees. Graph 3 shows the distribution of the sample by length of specialization, which was calculated based on 2013. This graph shows that 73.5% of the sample had completed their specialization in the last 10 years. It should be noted that the subjects who had two specializations were considered to have completed the oldest one. The gender distribution can be seen in Graph 4, with 67 (68.4%) women and 31 (31.6%) men.

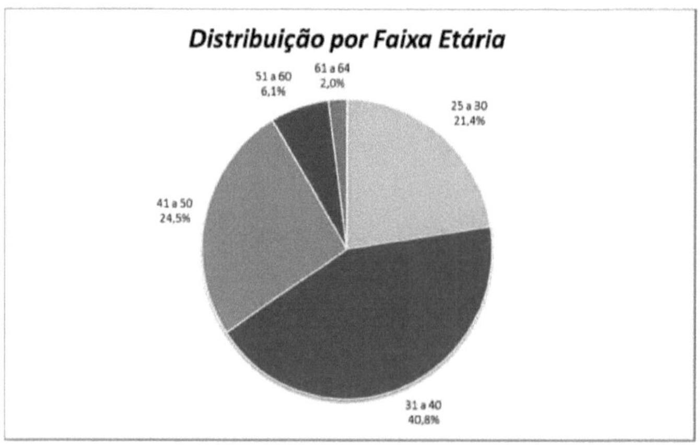

Graph 1: Distribution by age group

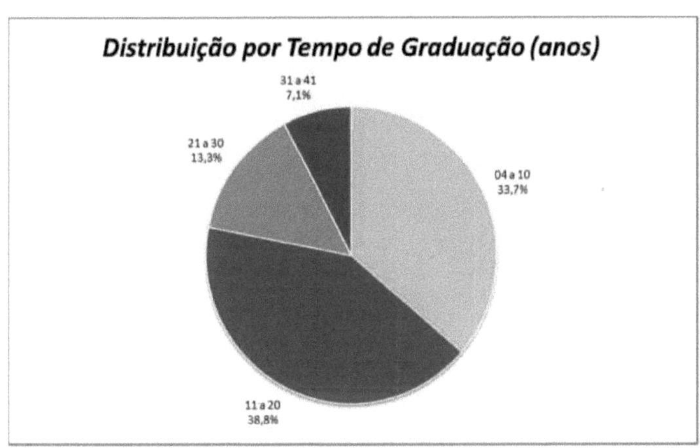

Graph 2: Distribution by Time since Graduation (years)

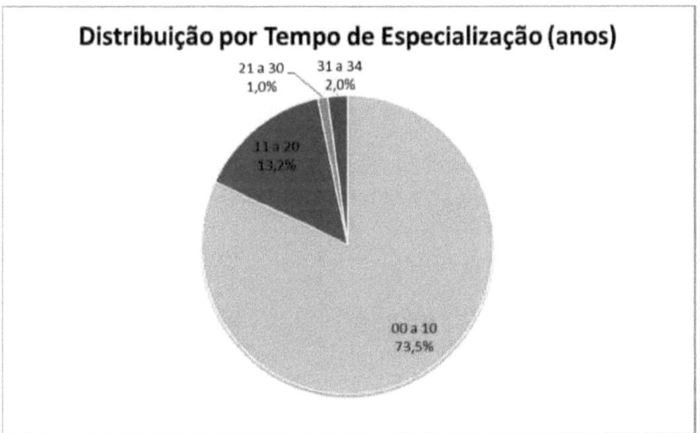

Graph 3: Distribution by length of specialization (years)

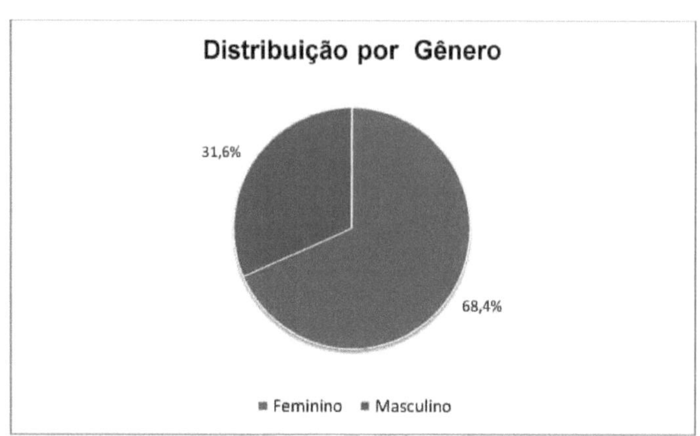

Graph 4: Distribution by gender

Graphs 5, 6, 7 and 8 show the distribution of responses from the sample studied in the areas of pathophysiology, psychophysiology, chronic pain and psychiatric disorders, respectively. The answers are broken down by item and the respective percentage figures. As mentioned above, the answers were grouped into "Disagree", when the item was answered between "0" and "3" on the scale; "Neutral", for "4", "5" and "6" on the scale; and "Agree", when the answer was between "7" and "10". In this part, the unanswered items were disregarded, which is why the percentage of some items does not add up to one hundred percent.

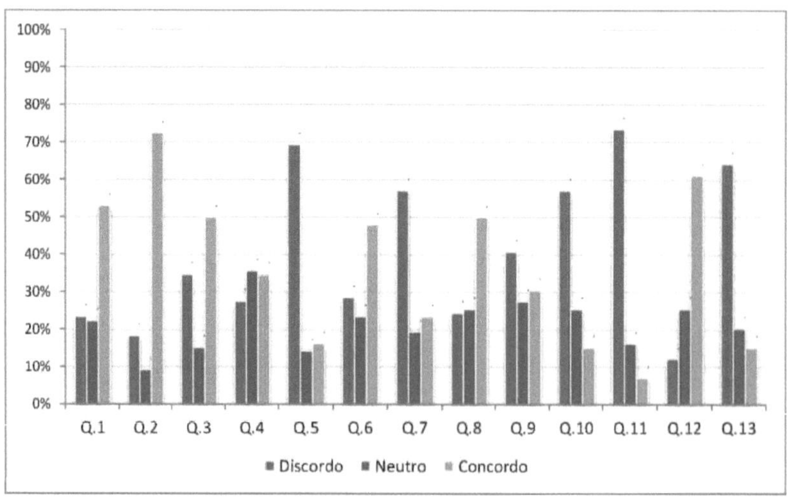

Graph 5: Frequency distribution of pathophysiology questions

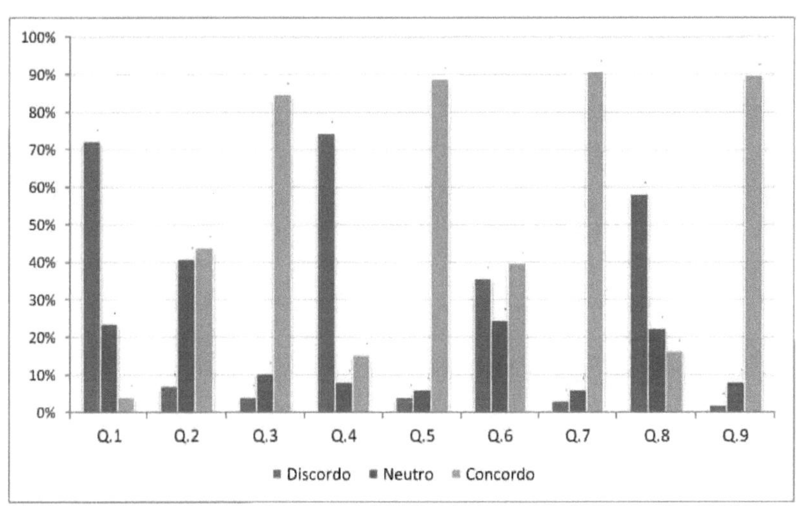

Graph 6: Frequency Distribution of Psychophysiology Questions

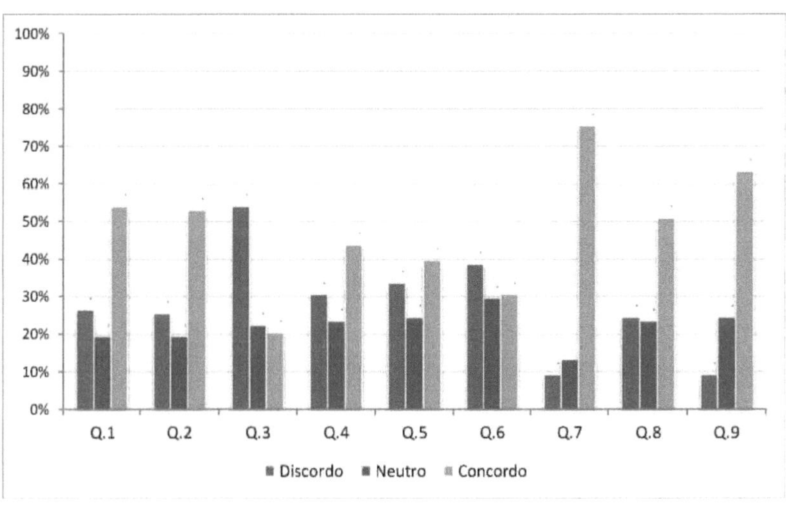

Graph 7: Frequency Distribution of Chronic Pain Questions

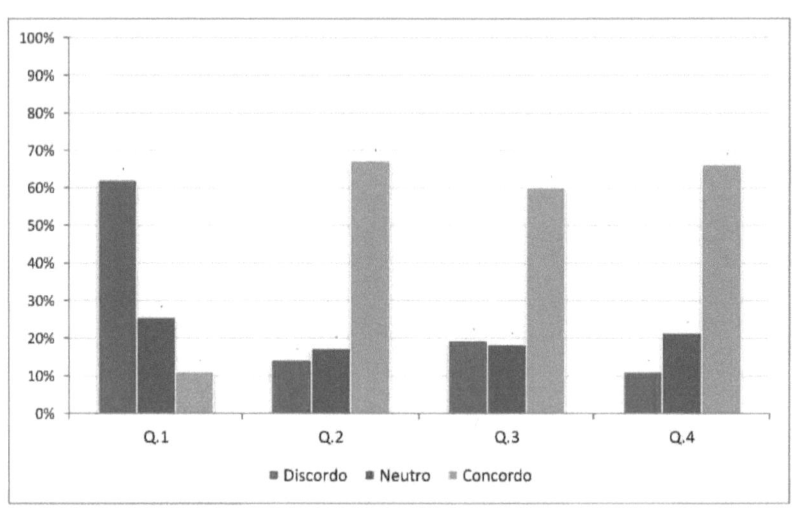

Graph 8: Frequency Distribution of Psychiatric Disorder Questions

Tables 1, 3, 5 and 7 then show the results of the responses for the areas of pathophysiology, psychophysiology, chronic pain and psychiatric disorders, taking into account the percentage of agreement between the studies that used the same questionnaire in the various cities where they were applied, and the experts' responses. And tables 2, 4, 6 and 8 are the p-values compared with the responses from the Manaus sample (reference). Remember that a p-value of less than 0.05 (significance level) is in red and indicates a statistically different result from the reference (Manaus) and, on the other hand, a p-value of more than 0.05 is in black and indicates a statistically similar result. In blue are p-values very close to the significance level.

Table 1: Distribution of papers by pathophysiology question

Pathophysiology		Manaus %	Experts %	Brasilia %	Kansas %	Seoul %	Seattle (Clinical) %	Seattle (Experts) %
Q.1 Disagree		23,5	85,0	14,5	10,0	26,0	11,3	23,5
Q.2	I disagree	18,4	85,0	12,3	26,0	28,5	29,9	43,2
Q.3	I disagree	34,7	77,0	19,6	19,0	36,5	14,4	34,6
Q.4	I disagree	27,6	100,0	47,8	52,0	38,5	48,5	72,3
Q.5	I disagree	69,4	92,0	62,3	28,0	54,5	28,5	50,0
Q.6	I disagree	28,6	85,0	50,7	33,0	59,5	31,8	47,1
Q.7	I disagree	57,1	77,0	64,5	49,0	54,0	32,8	67,1
Q.8	I disagree	24,5	77,0	32,6	32,0	24,5	24,5	40,3
Q.9	I disagree	40,8	92,0	60,9	46,0	41,0	40,3	66,9
Q.10	I disagree	57,1	92,0	59,4	- x-	49,5	45,3	42,9
Q.11	I disagree	73,5	85,0	71,7	33,0	48,0	42,6	48,3
Q.12	I agree	61,2	100,0	42,8	65,0	75,0	73,5	70,4
Q.13	I disagree	64,3	100,0	70,3	95,0	72,5	92,6	97,7

Table 2: P-values from table 1

Pathophysiology		Experts	Brasilia	Kansas	Seoul	Clinicians	Specialist
Q.1	I disagree	<0,001	0,078	0,005	0,815	0,005	0,960
Q.2	I disagree	<0,001	0,144	0,199	0,146	0,035	<0,001
Q.3	I disagree	0,003	0,009	0,006	0,909	<0,001	0,941
Q.4	I disagree	<0,001	0,002	<0,001	0,137	<0,001	<0,001
Q.5	I disagree	0,255	0,217	<0,001	0,037	<0,001	0,002
Q.6	I disagree	<0,001	<0,001	0,498	<0,001	0,580	0,003
Q.7	I disagree	0,172	0,253	0,216	0,674	<0,001	0,108
Q.8	I disagree	<0,001	0,216	0,219	0,902	0,985	0,010
Q.9	I disagree	0,003	0,002	0,475	0,997	0,892	<0,001
Q.10	I disagree	0,057	0,812	- x-	0,267	0,046	0,020
Q.11	I disagree	0,385	0,679	<0,001	<0,001	<0,001	<0,001
Q.12	I agree	0,006	0,005	0,583	0,055	0,035	0,129
Q.13	I disagree	0,009	0,331	<0,001	0,258	<0,001	<0,001

Table 3: Distribution of papers by question for psychophysiology

Psychophysiology	Manaus	Experts	Brasilia	Kansas	Seoul	Seattle (Clinicians)	Seattle (Experts)
	%	%	%	%	%	%	%
Q.1 Disagree	72,4	100,0	87,0	61,0	71,0	70,9	67,4
Q.2 Agree	43,9	77,0	52,9	53,0	59,5	50,0	58,4
Q.3 Agree	84,7	85,0	88,4	82,0	80,0	83,2	80,2
Q.4 Disagree	74,5	92,0	82,6	76,0	57,5	75,1	76,8
Q.5 Agree	88,8	100,0	93,5	90,0	59,5	91,2	89,4
Q.6 Agree	39,8	85,0	37,7	87,0	64,5	92,2	92,2
Q.7 Agree	90,8	100,0	91,3	81,0	74,0	77,7	82,2
Q.8 Disagree	58,2	85,0	62,3	57,0	74,0	61,6	62,4
Q.9 Agree	89,8%	92,0	90,6	88,0	69,0	88,2	89,9

Table 4: P-values from table 3

Psychophysiology		Experts	Brasilia	Kansas	Seoul	Clinicians	Specialist
Q.1	I disagree	0,030	0,005	0,069	0,695	0,757	0,335
Q.2	I agree	0,025	0,172	0,186	0,045	0,338	0,024
Q.3	I agree	0,994	0,509	0,542	0,326	0,698	0,344
Q.4	I disagree	0,424	0,171	0,795	0,013	0,978	0,667
Q.5	I agree	0,203	0,201	0,844	<0,001	0,594	0,965
Q.6	I agree	0,002	0,742	<0,001	0,001	<0,001	<0,001
Q.7	I agree	0,254	0,951	0,037	0,003	0,005	0,044
Q.8	I disagree	0,066	0,596	0,838	0,033	0,583	0,544
Q.9	I agree	0,572	0,841	0,673	<0,001	0,612	0,939

Table 5: Distribution of studies by question for chronic pain

Chronic Pain		Manaus	Experts	Brasilia	Kansas	Seoul	Seattle (Clinicians)	Seattle (Experts)
		%	%	%	%	%	%	%
Q.1	I disagree	26,5	85,0	30,4	27,0	46,5	23,3	25,1
Q.2	I disagree	25,5	93,0	30,4	46,0	42,0	41,7	55,9
Q.3	I disagree	54,1	89,0	61,6	65,0	46,5	50,0	61,8
Q.4	I disagree	30,6	100,0	50,7	70,0	63,0	69,7	80,2
Q.5	I agree	39,8	96,0	35,5	67,0	73,5	69,8	80,1
Q.6	I disagree	38,8	85,0	63,8	66,0	65,5	62,4	68,0
Q.7	I agree	75,5	96,0	66,7	79,0	74,0	69,0	74,0
Q.8	I agree	51,0	89,0	57,2	61,0	64,5	67,8	68,2
Q.9	I agree	63,3	89,0	71,0	67,0	66,5	80,2	82,6

Table 6: P-values from table 5

Chronic Pain		Experts	Brasilia	Kansas	Seoul	Clinicians	Specialist
Q.1	I disagree	<0,001	0,593	0,982	0,007	0,493	0,760
Q.2	I disagree	<0,001	0,479	0,002	0,032	0,007	<0,001
Q.3	I disagree	<0,001	0,248	0,105	0,293	0,481	0,241
Q.4	I disagree	<0,001	0,003	<0,001	<0,001	<0,001	<0,001
Q.5	I agree	<0,001	0,431	<0,001	<0,001	<0,001	<0,001
Q.6	I disagree	<0,001	<0,001	<0,001	<0,001	<0,001	<0,001
Q.7	I agree	0,053	0,143	0,610	0,783	0,227	0,712
Q.8	I agree	<0,001	0,403	0,144	0,076	0,006	0,005
Q.9	I agree	0,011	0,257	0,626	0,730	0,002	<0,001

Table 7: Distribution of papers by question for psychiatric disorders

Psychiatric disorders		Manaus	Experts	Brasilia	Kansas	Seoul	Seattle (Clinicians)	Seattle (Experts)
		%	%	%	%	%	%	%
Q.1	I disagree	62,2	100,0	66,7	69,0	61,5	57,5	73,9
Q.2	I agree	67,3	86,0	64,5	73,0	66,5	57,4	72,6
Q.3	I agree	60,2	79,0	65,9	60,0	73,5	56,2	64,6
Q.4	I agree	66,3	79,0	62,3	83,0	66,5	79,4	78,8

Table 8: P-values from table 7

Psychiatric disorders		Experts	Brasilia	Kansas	Seoul	Clinicians	Specialist
Q.1	I disagree	0,005	0,483	0,305	0,817	0,438	0,052
Q.2	I agree	0,162	0,649	0,376	0,829	0,087	0,379
Q.3	I agree	0,184	0,431	0,975	0,094	0,499	0,522
Q.4	I agree	0,359	0,457	0,006	0,941	0,017	0,027

Graphs 9 to 43 are a comparison of all the answers, question by question and compared with the experts and other similar works. In blue, in the first bar, are the answers from the experts, in yellow are the answers from Manaus and from all the papers with statistically similar results and in gray those with statistically different answers from the Manaus sample. The values in the bars are the p-values always compared to the response of the Manaus sample, the study's reference (ref).

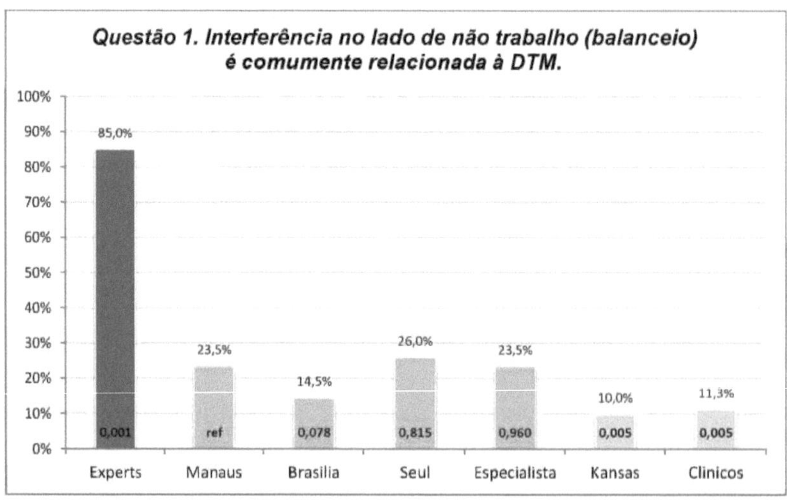

Graph 9: Distribution of Papers on Question 1 (Disagree) of Pathophysiology

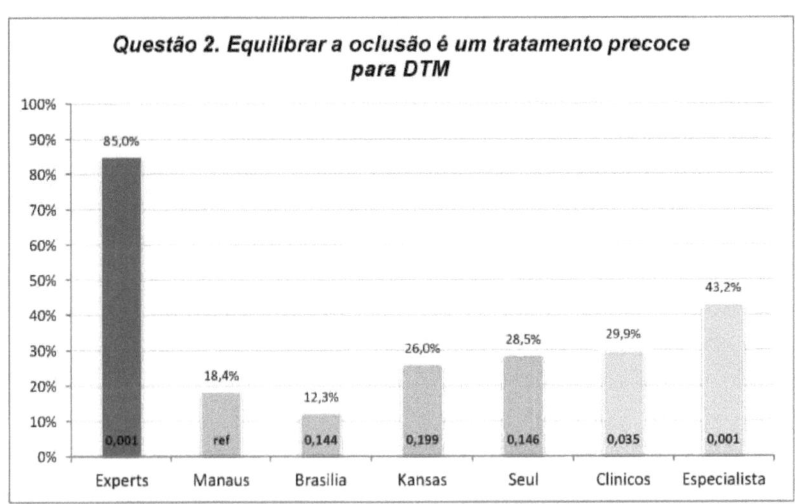

Graph 10: Distribution of Papers on Question 2 (Disagree) of Pathophysiology

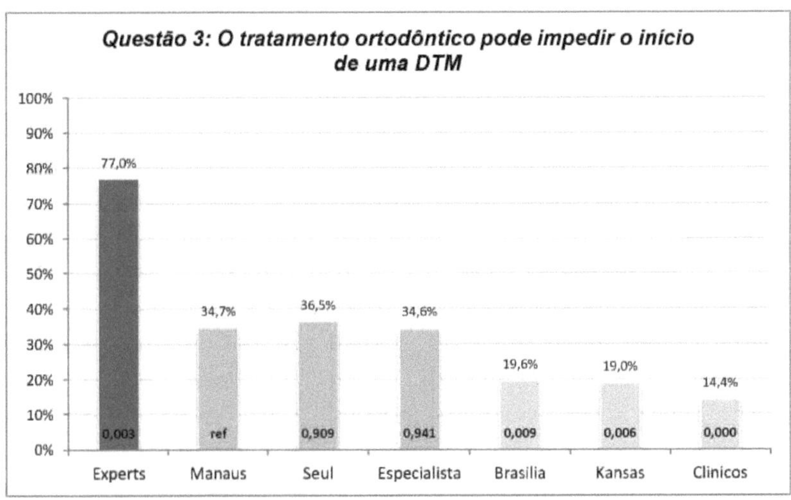

Graph 11: Distribution of Papers on Question 3 (Disagree) of Pathophysiology

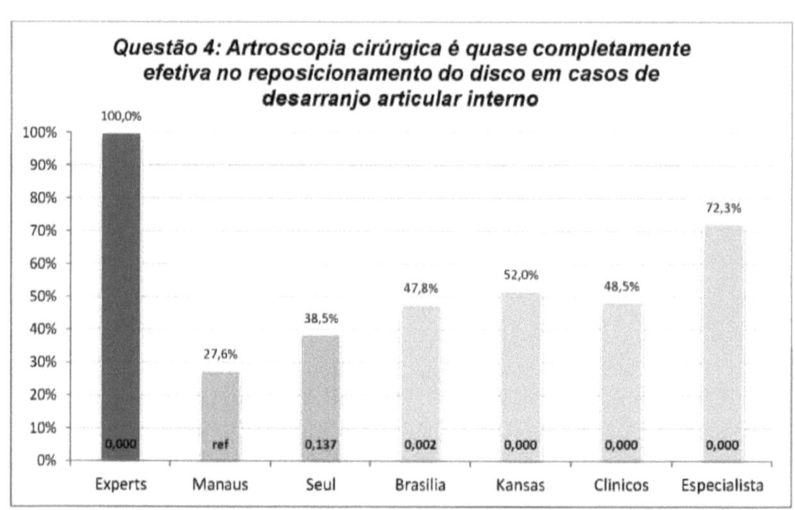

Graph 12: Distribution of Papers on Question 4 (Disagree) of Pathophysiology

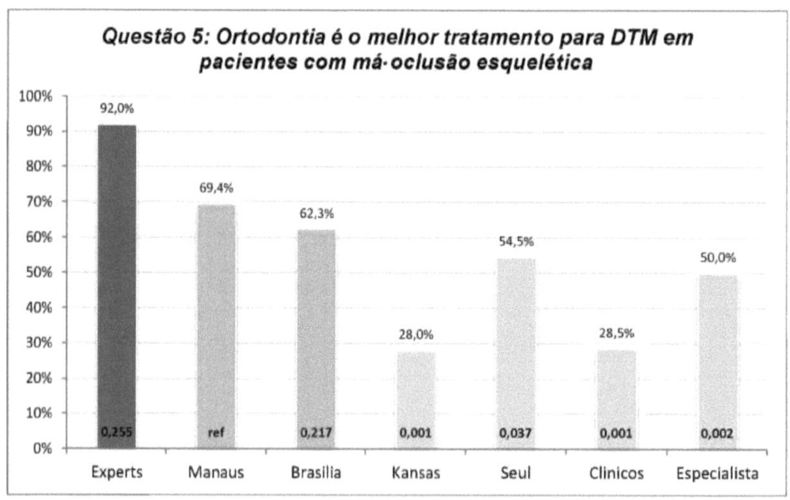

Graph 13: Distribution of Works on Question 5 (Disagree) of Pathophysiology

34

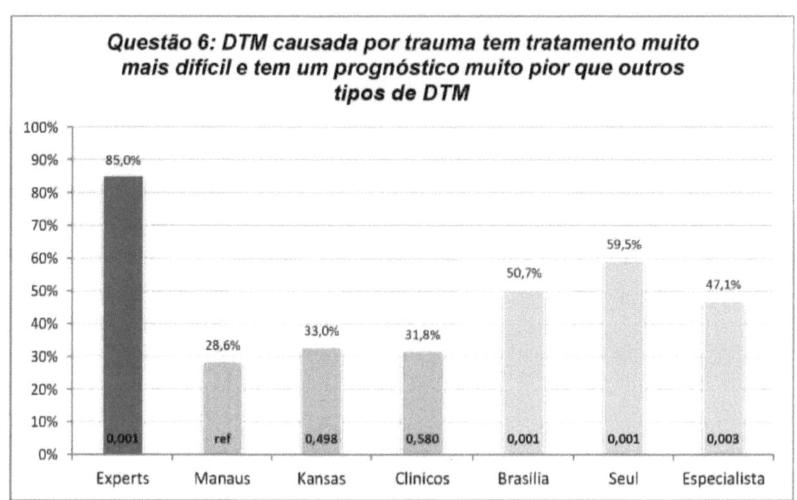

Graph 14: Distribution of Papers on Question 6 (Disagree) of Pathophysiology

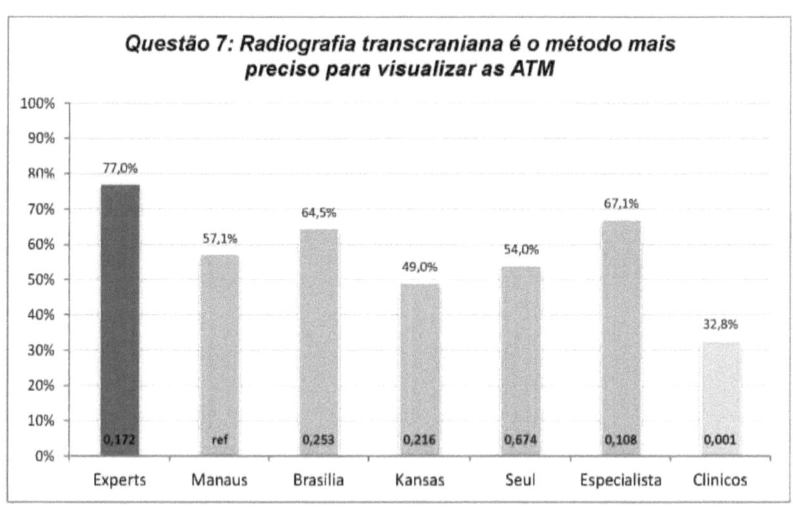

Graph 15: Distribution of Papers on Question 7 (Disagree) of Pathophysiology

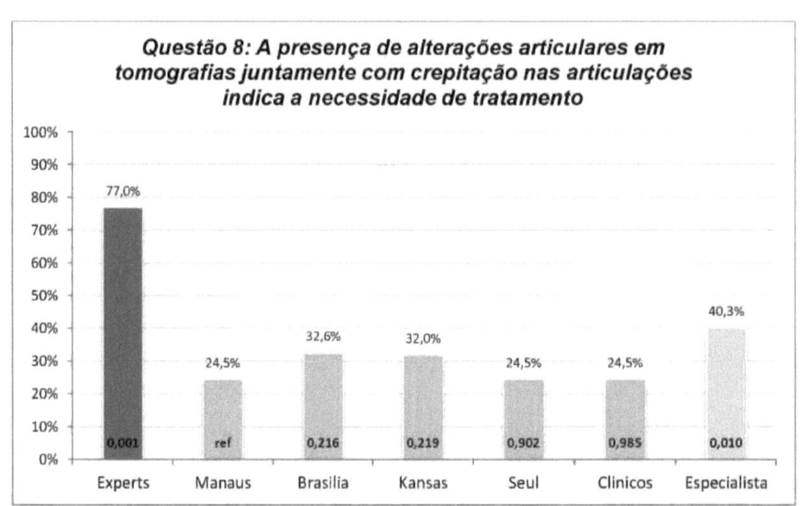

Graph 16: Distribution of Papers on Question 8 (Disagree) of Pathophysiology

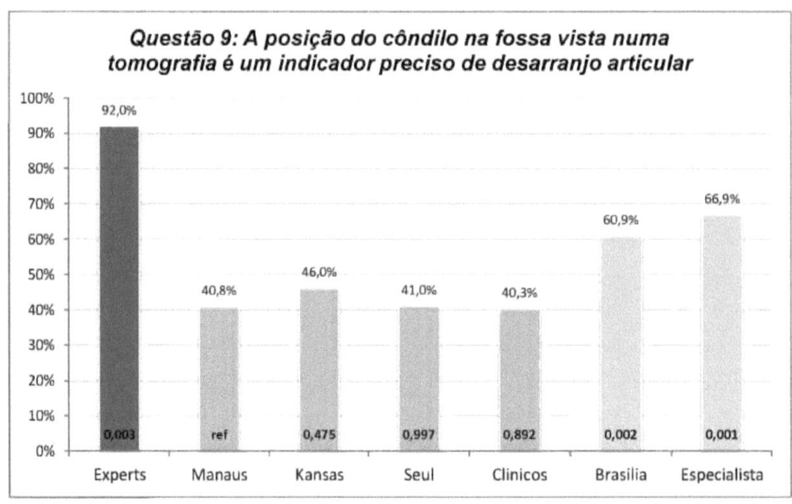

Graph 17: Distribution of Papers on Question 9 (Disagree) of Pathophysiology

36

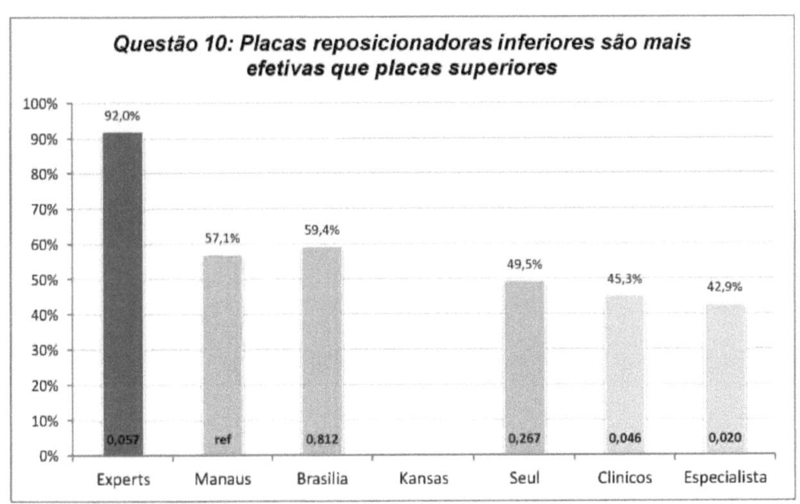

Graph 18: Distribution of Papers on Question 10 (Disagree) of Pathophysiology

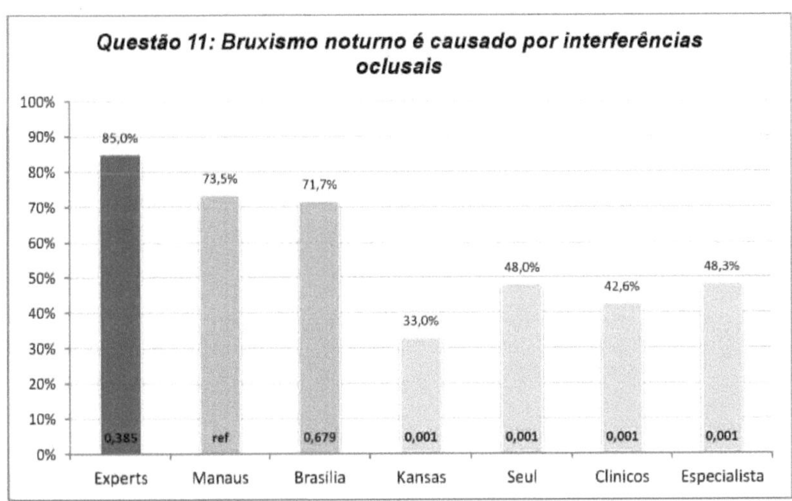

Graph 19: Distribution of Papers on Question 11 (Disagree) of Pathophysiology

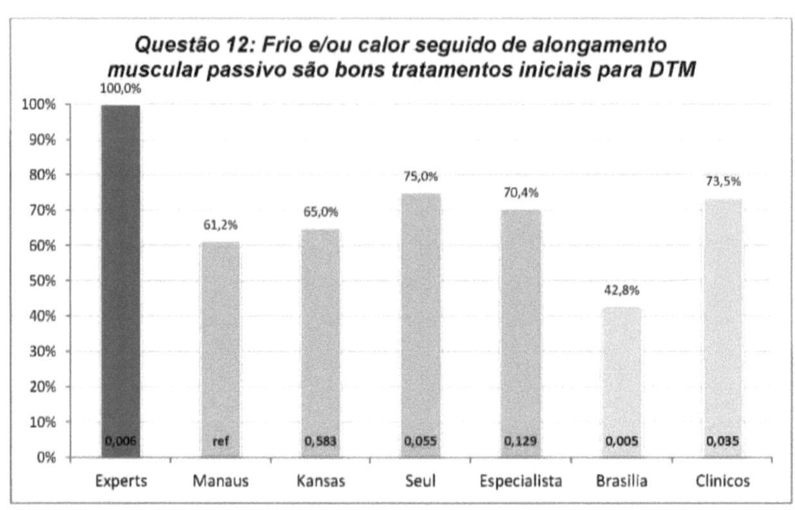

Graph 20: Distribution of Papers on Question 12 (Agree) of Pathophysiology

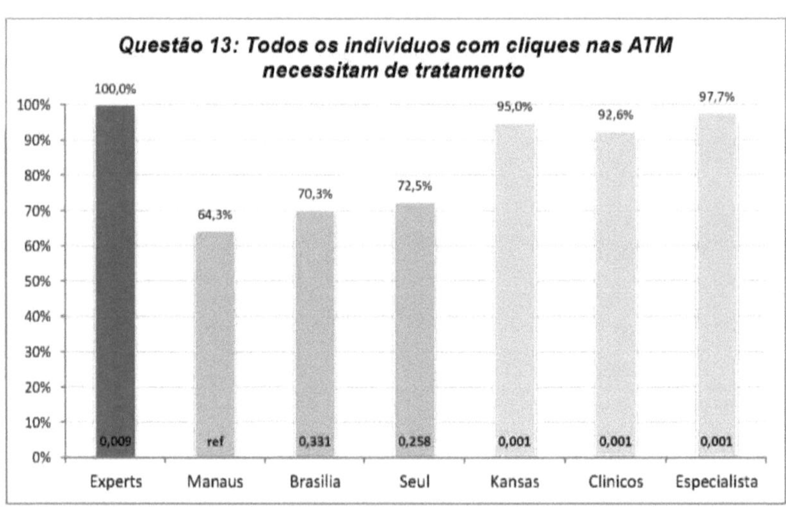

Graph 21: Distribution of Papers on Question 13 (Disagree) of Pathophysiology

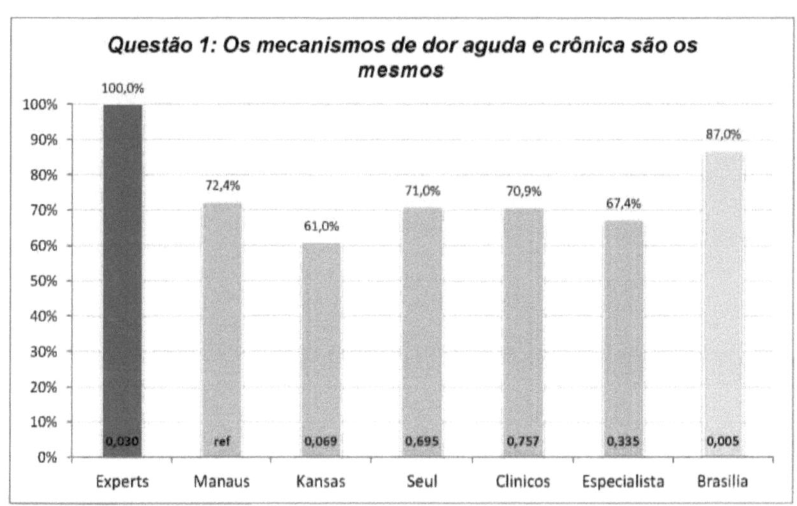

Graph 22: Distribution of Papers on Question 1 (Disagree) of Psychophysiology

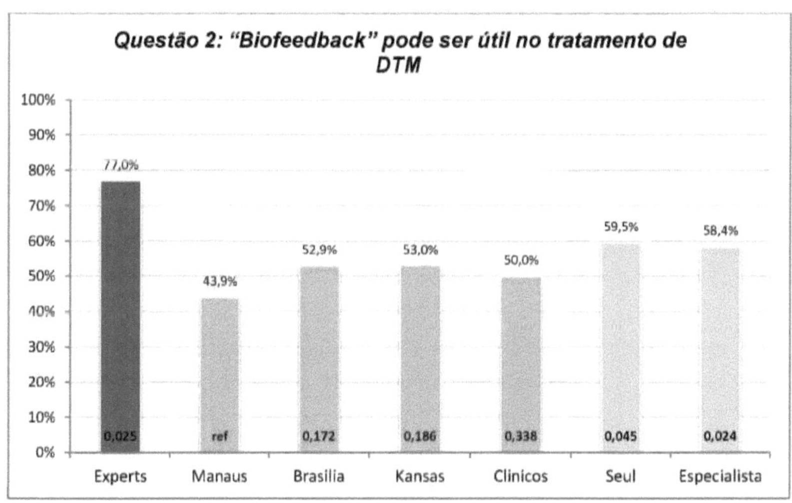

Graph 23: Distribution of Papers on Psychophysiology Question 2 (Agree)

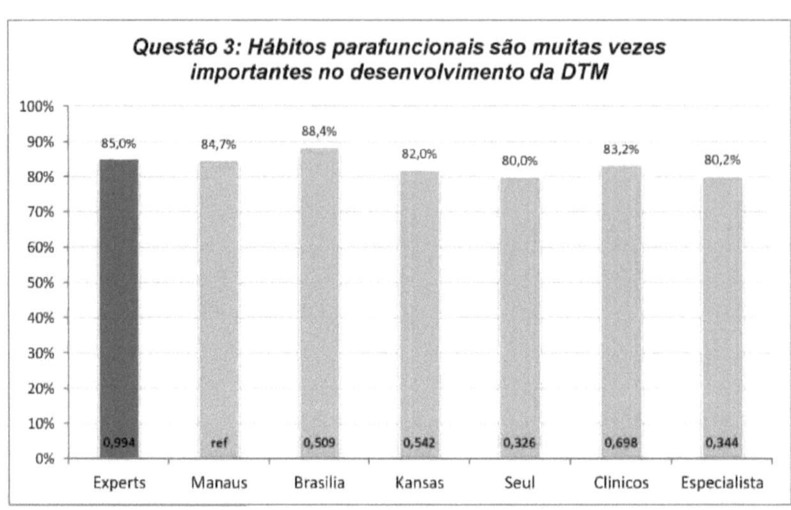

Graph 24: Distribution of Papers on Question 3 (Agree) of Psychophysiology

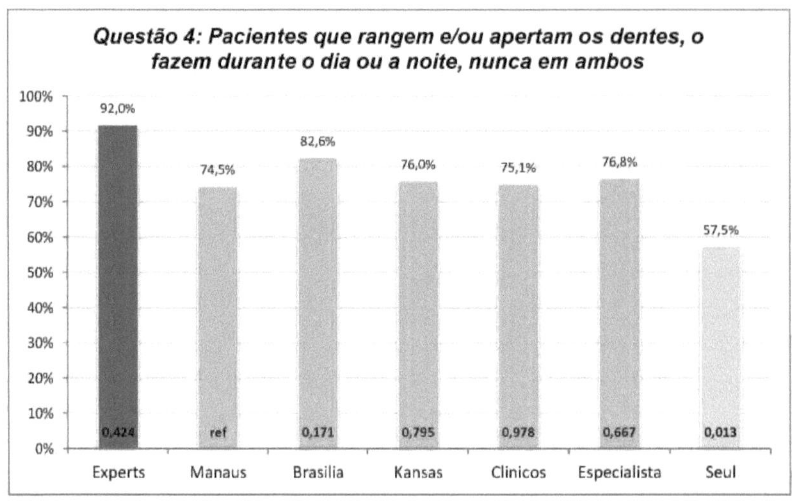

Graph 25: Distribution of Papers on Question 4 (Disagree) in Psychophysiology

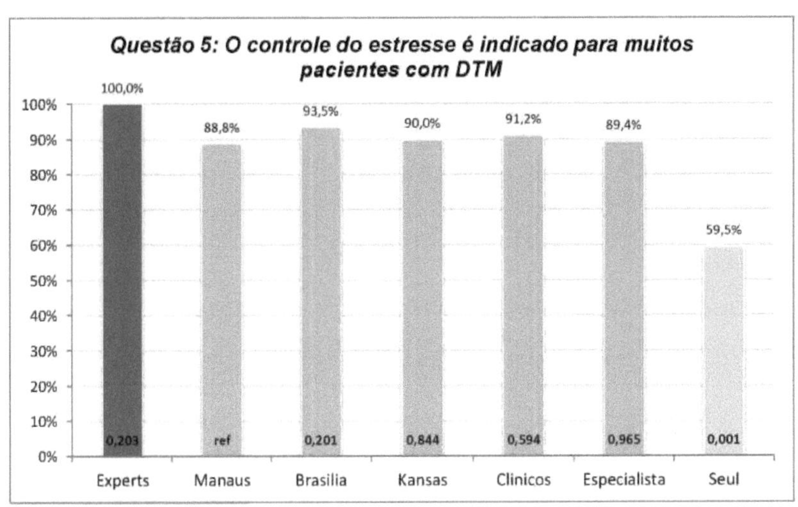

Graph 26: Distribution of Papers on Question 5 (Agree) of Psychophysiology

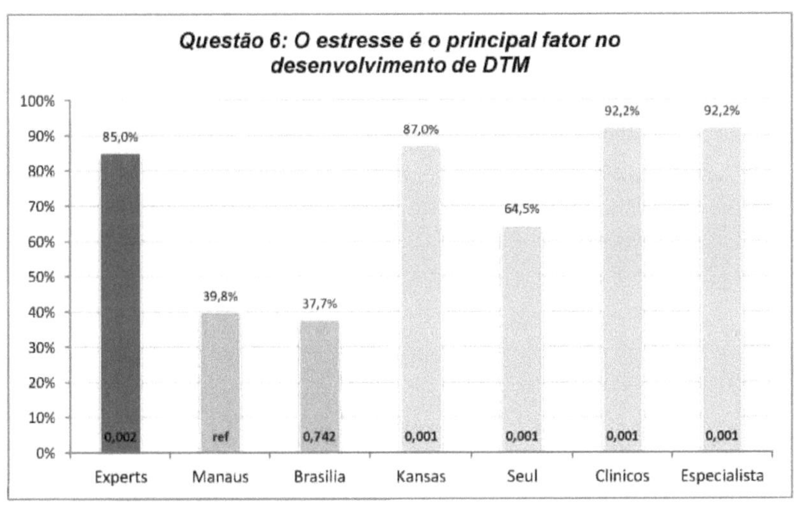

Graph 27: Distribution of Papers on Psychophysiology Question 6 (Agree)

41

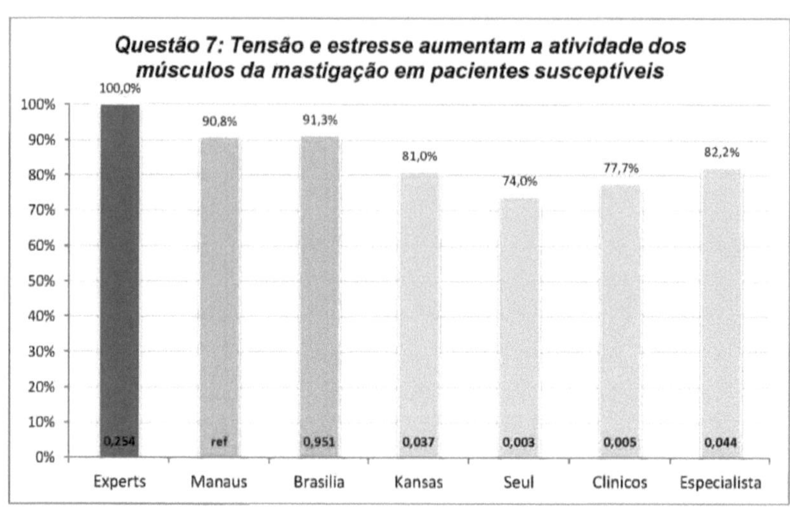

Graph 28: Distribution of Papers on Psychophysiology Question 7 (Agree)

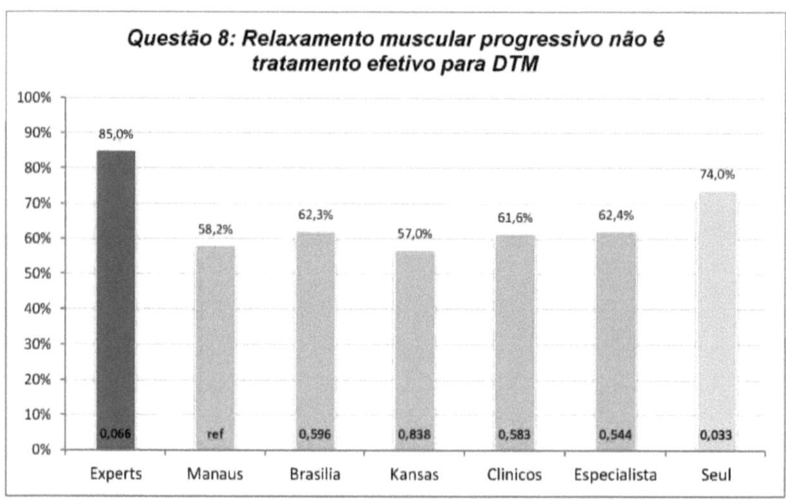

Graph 29: Distribution of Papers on Question 8 (Disagree) in Psychophysiology

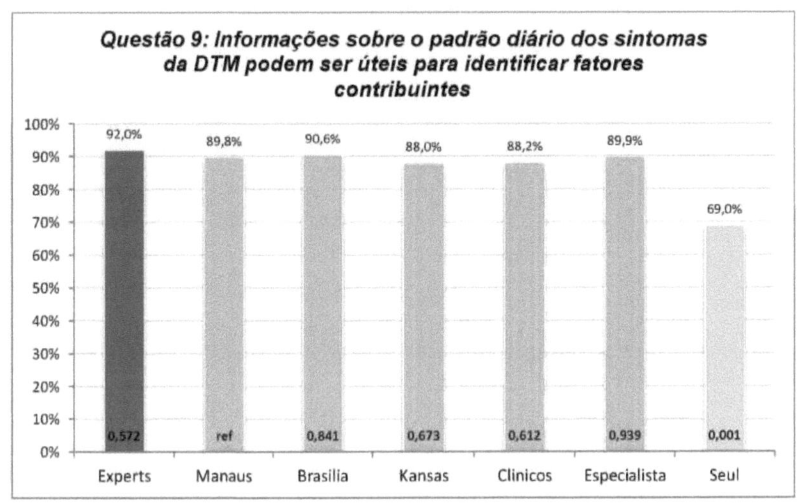

Graph 30: Distribution of Papers on Question 9 (Agree) of Psychophysiology

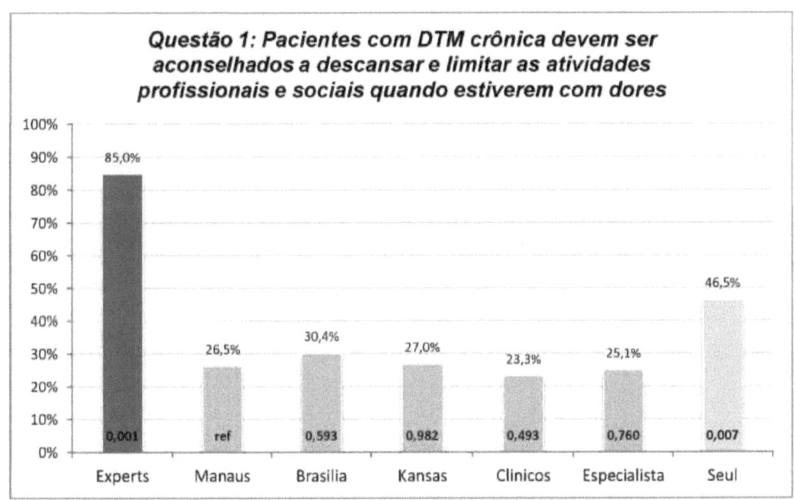

Graph 31: Distribution of Works on Chronic Pain Question 1 (Disagree)

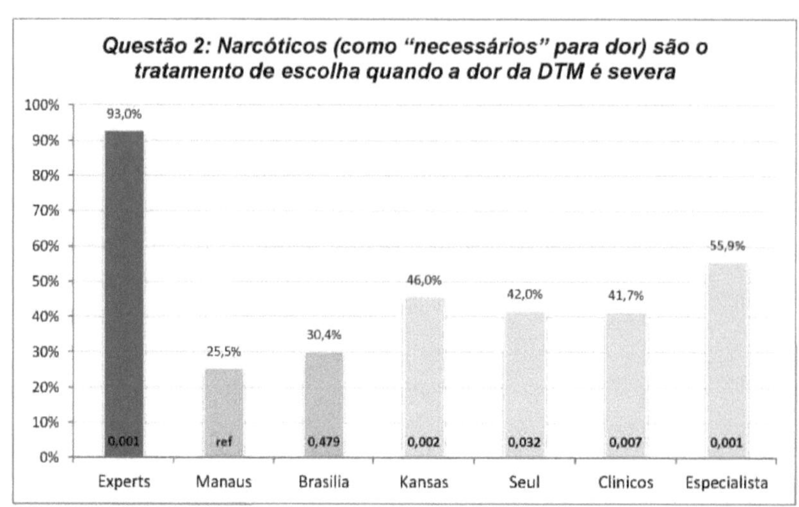

Graph 32: Distribution of Works on Question 2 (Disagree) of Chronic Pain

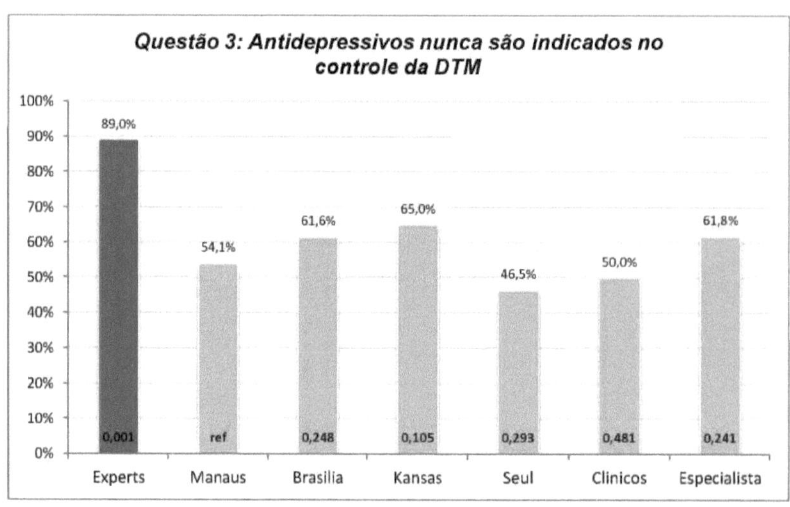

Graph 33: Distribution of Works on Chronic Pain Question 3 (Disagree)

44

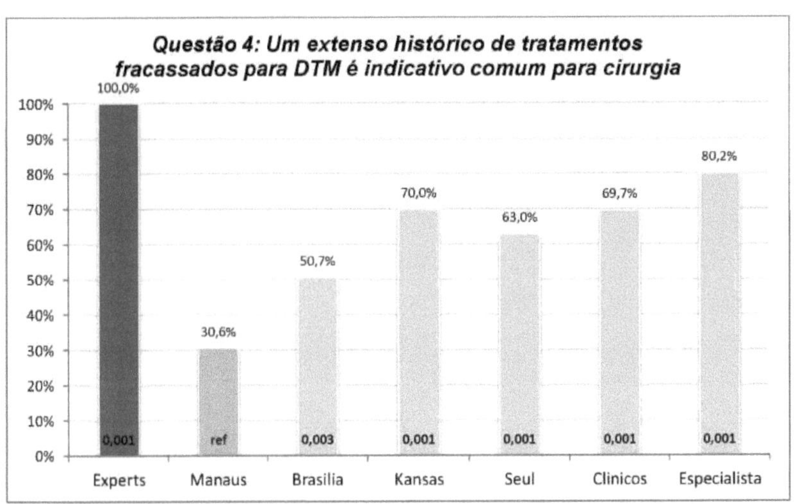

Graph 34: Distribution of Works on Question 4 (Disagree) of Chronic Pain

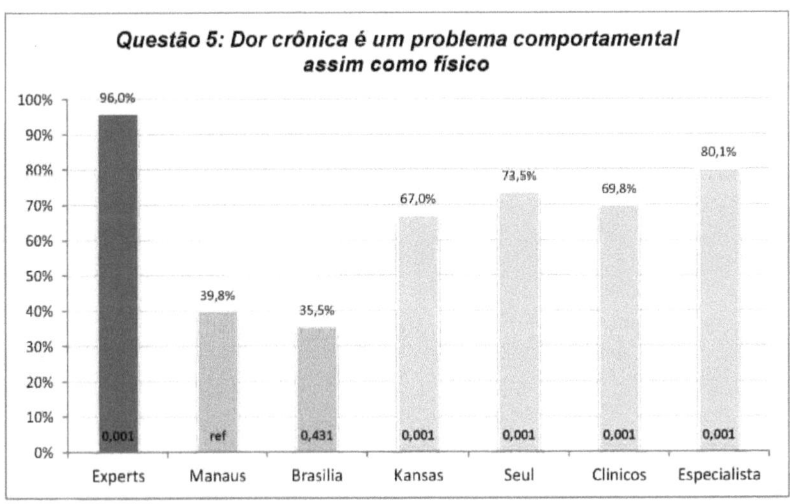

Graph 35: Distribution of Works on Chronic Pain Question 5 (Agree)

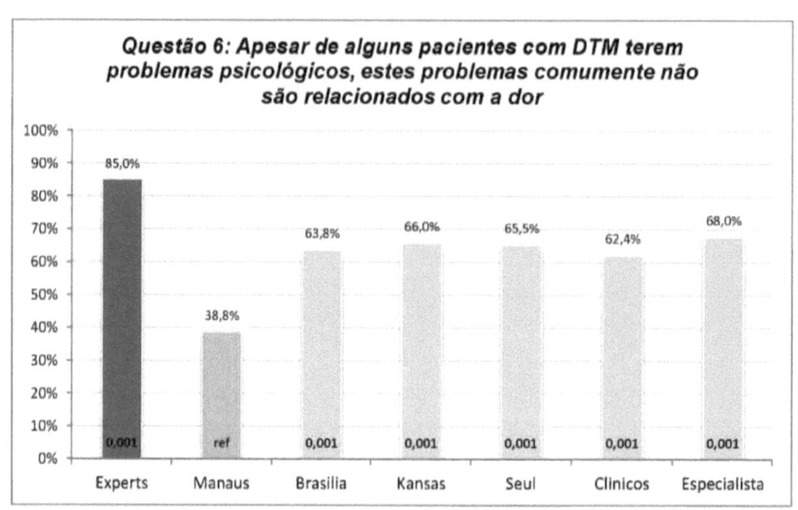

Graph 36: Distribution of Works on Chronic Pain Question 6 (Disagree)

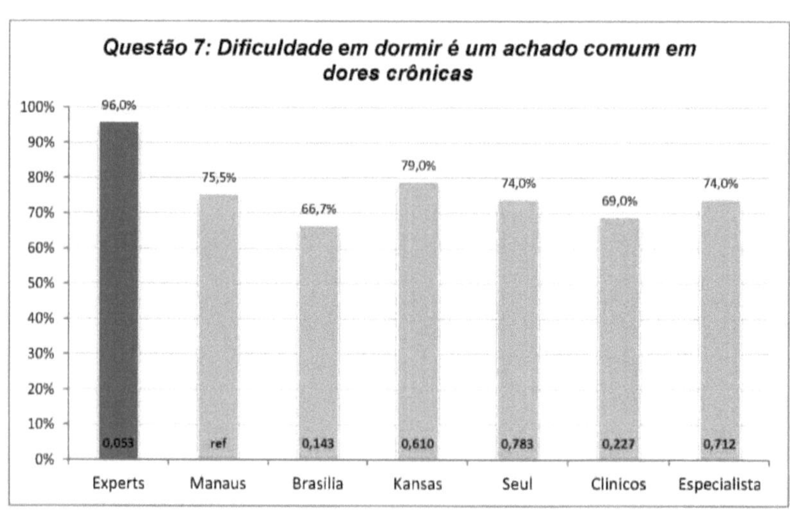

Graph 37: Distribution of Works on Chronic Pain Question 7 (Agree)

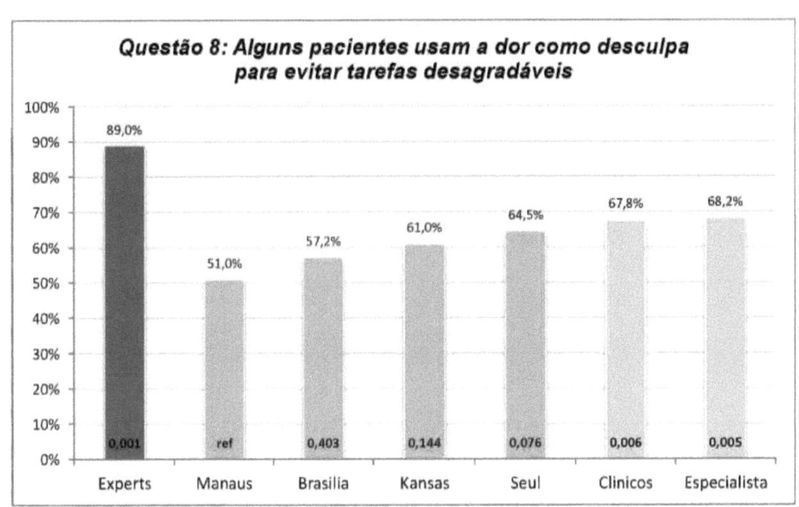

Graph 38: Distribution of Works on Chronic Pain Question 8 (Agree)

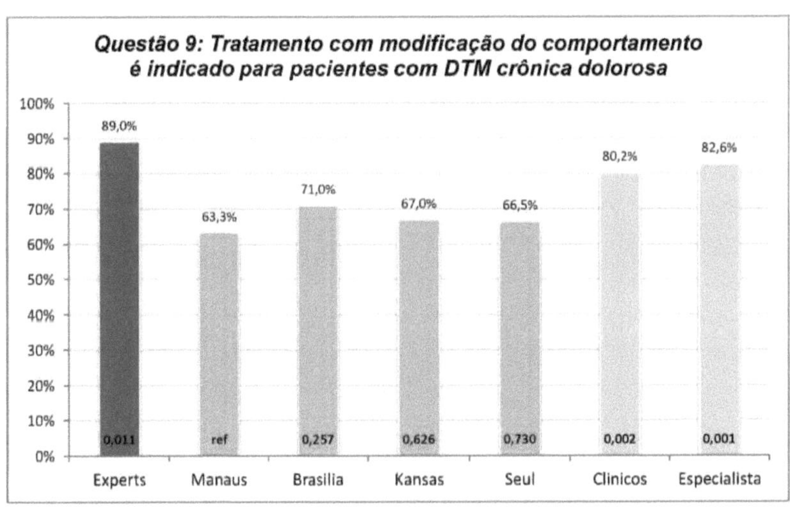

Graph 39: Distribution of Works on Chronic Pain Question 9 (Agree)

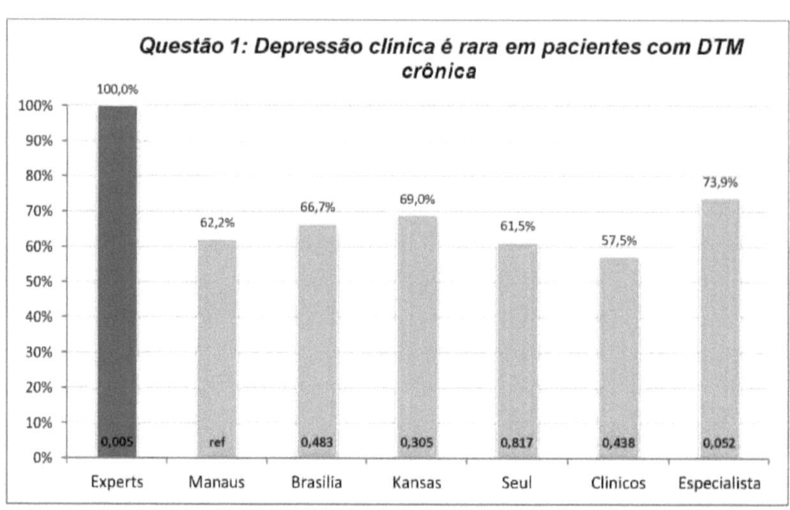

Graph 40: Distribution of Papers on Question 1 (Disagree) of Psychiatric Disorders

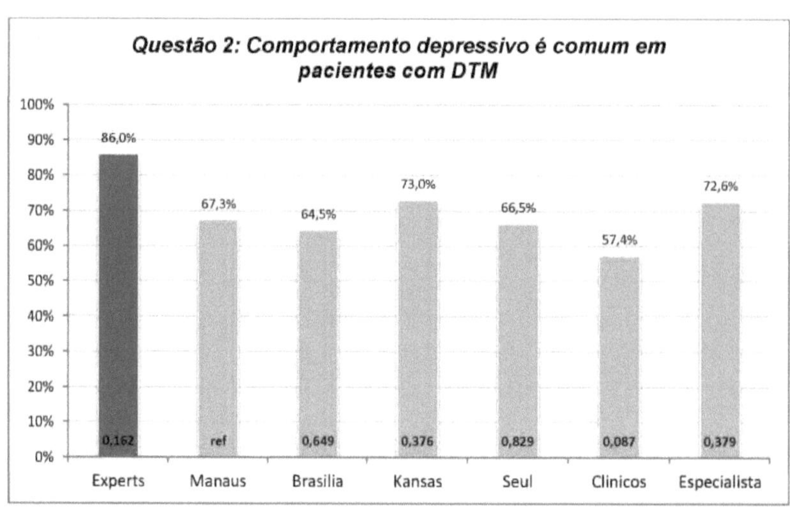

Graph 41: Distribution of Papers on Question 2 (Agree) Psychiatric Disorders

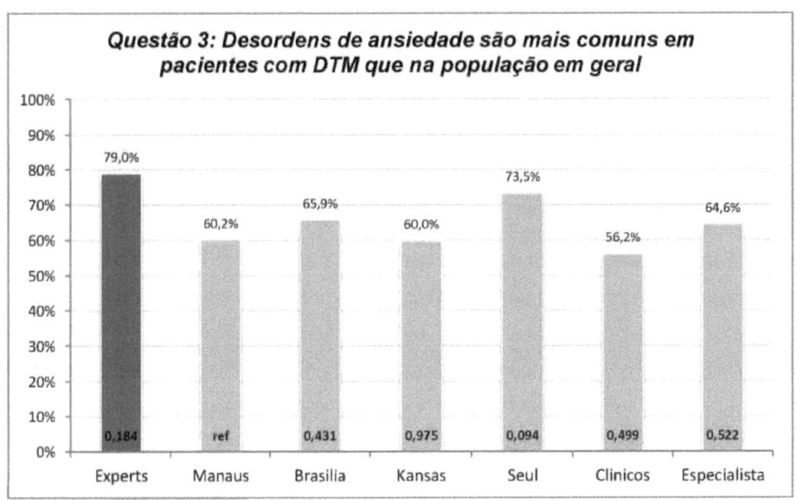

Graph 42: Distribution of Papers on Question 3 (Agree) of Psychiatric Disorders

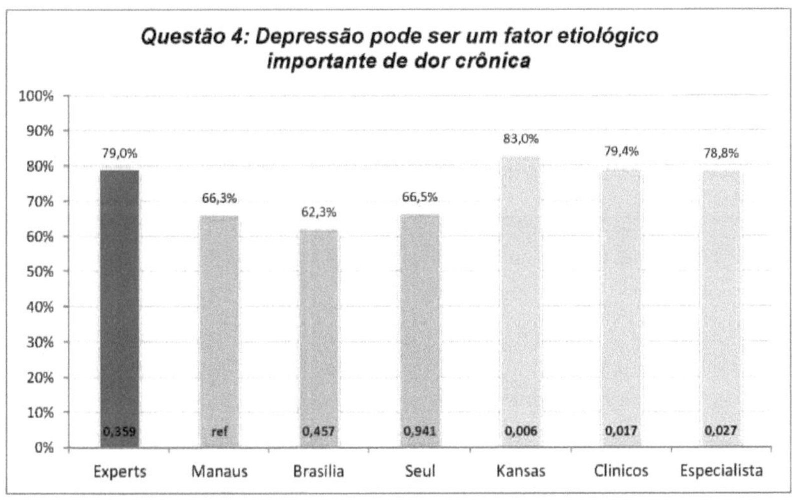

Graph 43: Distribution of Papers on Question 4 (Agree) Psychiatric Disorders

6   Discussion

In this study, as in all studies involving data collection, the findings are specific to the sample of orthodontists and/or functional jaw orthopedists in the state of Amazonas and the period studied, and therefore should not be extrapolated to other populations. This recommendation was also cited in articles on the Seattle (Le Resche et al., 1993), Kansas (Glaros et al., 1994), Seoul (Lee et al., 2000) and Brasilia (Ribeiro, 2009) studies.

Data collection for this study took place between January 2012 and February 2013. The studies used as a reference for comparing the results of this study had their data collection phase between June and September 1990 (Le Resche et al., 1993), May and June 1991 (Glaros et al., 1994), during 1996 (Lee et al., 2000) and between August and October 2006 (Ribeiro, 2009). It is therefore clear that comparing the responses of professionals from the same field of knowledge in different periods and locations can lead to a misinterpretation of the data. It should be borne in mind that knowledge about the various aspects of TMD can change due to the evolution of scientific methods and acquired knowledge (McNeill, 1997a; Venâncio, Camparis, 2002; Forssell, Kalso, 2004).

During the bibliographic survey of this work, four articles and one master's thesis were found in the databases searched that related questionnaires and TMD in Brazil.

The first looked at dental surgeons' knowledge of the etiology, incidence and diagnosis of TMD (Francesquini Jr. et al., 1999), and started off with a mistake in the title of the paper, as the word incidence should have read prevalence. Furthermore, the methodology was confusing, the questionnaire was not clearly disclosed and the correct answers did not appear in the article.

The second only described the use of a questionnaire to screen patients for possible TMD (Manfredi et al., 2001), while the third set out to assess the knowledge of DCs in the field of TMD (Venâncio, Camparis, 2002). However, this last study had an unclear methodology regarding the creation of the questionnaire, the size of the sample and the reference for evaluating the answers obtained. This survey, carried out with dentists in the city of Ribeirão Preto, in the state of São Paulo, led the authors to conclude, in 2002, that the concepts of TMD diagnosis and treatment did not yet have the desired scientific support, which contradicts the scientific literature published until then (McNeill, 1997a).

The fourth article surveyed the attitudes and beliefs of orthodontists with regard to TMD/OFD (Moana Filho, 2005). This is a good article, with a clear methodology and a questionnaire based on previously published articles. However, it doesn't provide answers to the technical-scientific questions, which makes it impossible to assess orthodontists' knowledge, which is the aim of this study.

The aim of the study was to assess the knowledge of dental surgeons in Brasilia about TMD (Ribeiro, 2009). There was a clear methodology, a questionnaire validated for Portuguese and replicated from an American study that had already been carried out in three other studies. It was therefore chosen as the basis for this study and for comparing the data collected in Amazonas with the consensus of TMD experts and with the samples obtained in other cities, even if they were not recent.

6.1 Sample characteristics

The sample obtained in the state of Amazonas, sometimes referred to as Manaus because only 1 interviewee did not work in the city, had a mean age of 37.9 years, older than the sample from Brasilia (Ribeiro, 2009) and younger than the samples from Seattle (Le Resche et al., 1993) and Kansas (Glaros et al., 1994). The average age of respondents in Brasilia was 31.2 years, while in Seattle it was 45 years for general practitioners and 48 years for specialists. In Kansas, the average age of respondents was 44 for general practitioners and 48 for specialists. There are two possible explanations for this difference: either the dentists in Brasilia are simply younger, or there were differences in the way the data was collected and where the dentists were approached. It should also be noted that the Korean article by Lee et al. (2000) did not describe the age of the sample.

With regard to predominant gender, in Manaus the majority of orthodontists and/or functional jaw orthopedists are women, 68.4% compared to only 31.6% of men. This data agrees with the sample of dental surgeons in Brasilia and disagrees with the figures found in similar studies where there is a significant majority of male respondents. In Brasilia (Ribeiro, 2009), for example, just over 41% of the dentists surveyed were male, while in Seattle (Le Resche et al., 1993) and Kansas (Glaros et al., 1994) they were over 90%. In the Seoul study (Lee et al., 2000) it was only mentioned that the majority were male.

The average length of specialization of the sample from the state of Amazonas was 6.44 years with a standard deviation of 1.36 years, ranging from recent specialists to orthodontists with 34 years' experience.

6.2 Questionnaire

The questionnaire was developed at the University of Washington and was used to collect data in the cities of Seattle, Kansas, Seoul, Brasilia and as the basis for a study in Ostergotland, Vastmanland and Gothenburg in Sweden. An important point in the creation of the questionnaire was the inclusion only of statements that obtained more than 75% of "agree" or "disagree" answers from the group called experts, as already described in the methodology of this work.

Although Glaros et al. (1994) and Lee et al. (2000) used the same questionnaire and methodology in their work, some differences are worth noting. In Glaros et al. (1994), in the section on chronic pain, there are 10 items, while in the original questionnaire there are only nine statements in this area. Furthermore, the item "To determine when TMD is chronic, the only important factor is the time elapsed since the onset of symptoms" is not found in the original article by Le Resche et al. (1993). Furthermore, in the section on pathophysiology, it can be seen that the original questionnaire contains 13 items, unlike the 1994 article, which contains only 12 statements. Lastly, the item "Lower repositioning plates are more effective than upper plates" was not included in this study.

On the other hand, in the article by Lee et al. (2000), the response to the item "Progressive muscle relaxation is not an effective treatment for TMD", included in the TMD psychophysiology section, the consensus of the experts in the original article was "disagree" with 82% agreement. However, in the Korean article, the authors cited "agree" as the consensus among the experts, also with 82% agreement. Therefore, the interviewees' response was compared in that article with a different reference to the one cited in the original article. It is possible that this is just a graphical error, but as there is no certification of this, the comparison of the Manaus sample with the Seoul responses may be invalid from a methodological point of view.

Tegelberg et al. (2007), formulated a 37-question questionnaire based on the Seattle questionnaire, but made some modifications to adapt it to the subject of TMD in adolescents and children, such as: excluding some questions, adding some and changing the wording of others. In addition, another expert group of 19 TMD specialists from Sweden, who are members of the Swedish Academy of Temporomandibular Disorders and have published extensively. Comparison with the Manaus data would be invalid, as some questions were changed. However, this study served to compare the responses of the Seattle experts in 1990 with the Swedish experts in 2005. This is discussed in the concluding remarks.

6.3 Discussion of results

Comparing data as a parameter makes it possible to discuss this data qualitatively. On the other hand, simply describing the data in a study is only conducive to demonstrating the results, making the work qualitatively limited. The main aim of this study was to situate the opinions of orthodontists in Manaus in relation to the consensus of researchers in the field and thus to provide data in a context which would allow us to show how close the responses of the sample were to those of researchers in the field. To this end, we tried to replicate as precisely as possible the methodology and statistical analysis of the data described in the work by Le Resche et al. (1993).

The disagreements between the answers given by the Manaus orthodontists and those given by the experts can be explained in two ways: either they simply disagreed with the opinion of the experts on the questionnaire items, or they were uncertain and lacked knowledge about the issues raised. This point of view was also mentioned in the original article (Le Resche et al., 1993) and was part of the methodology used to evaluate the results obtained in Seattle. This may indicate the low quality of the education acquired by the sample.

6.3.1 Pathophysiology

This group of questions assesses the respondents' knowledge of the biomedical and biomechanical aspects of TMD, namely occlusion, orthodontics as treatment and prevention, imaging tests and TMD treatment. The results of this study showed that there was considerable divergence in the opinions of the interviewees from Manaus and the experts. There was significant agreement on only 3 of the 13 items, questions 5, 7 and 11. The three questions deal with non-controversial topics, orthodontics as a treatment for TMD, transcranial radiography as an accurate method of visualizing TMJ and Bruxism being caused by occlusal interferences.

Graph 5 shows the frequency distribution of the answers given by the Amazonians to the pathophysiology questions and Table 1 compares the answers given by the consensus of experts with those given by other studies. Graphs 9 to 21 also show the individual responses to each question.

The first three questions deal with occlusal issues, "interference on the non-working side (balancing) is commonly related to TMD", "balancing occlusion is an early treatment for TMD" and "orthodontic treatment can prevent the onset of TMD". According to a literature review, the presence of malocclusion, as well as its treatment, does not prevent, establish or cure TMD (Just et al., 1991; Luther, 1998b; Michelotti, Iodice, 2010), which was corroborated by the TMD experts when they widely disagreed with these statements. However, Amazonians still believe in the occlusion factor as an etiological agent for TMD, a concept introduced by James Costen in 1934, since 53% of respondents agreed with the first item, 72.4% with the second and 50% agreed with the third statement. It is necessary to disseminate this knowledge, since in other studies too, disagreement with these statements was extremely low.

Forsell et al. (1999) rightly reported that probably many dentists around the world still believed occlusal factors to be very important in the development of TMD, and consequently also considered occlusal treatment to be essential in the management of TMD patients. According to Forsell & Kalso (2004), it was difficult to convince dentists who believed in the influence of occlusion on TMD that this influence was non-existent or very small. This issue will probably only be resolved when DCs believe in evidence-based medicine.

Question 4, "Surgical arthroscopy is almost completely effective in repositioning the disc in cases of internal articular derangement", had unanimous disagreement by the consensus, while in Manaus, the interviewees showed doubt as there was no statistically significant difference between agree, neutral and disagree. However, the Seoul sample had a statistically similar result, and all the other samples disagreed by up to 52%, with the exception of the Seattle experts who disagreed by 77%. This result may indicate a lack of information about the indication of this surgical procedure or even a lack of knowledge about it, which, because it is an invasive technique and is performed under general anesthesia involving cannulas, trocars, a tiny arthroscope connected to a camera system that projects the maximized image onto a monitor, requires the surgeon to be skilled and experienced (Grossman, Grossman, 2011).

Respondents would need to remember or be aware of a simple premise that TMD treatment should be as cost-effective and reversible as possible (Le Resche et al., 1993; Glaros et al., 1994; Lee et al., 2000). In addition, guidelines recommend avoiding the treatment of asymptomatic clicks, as they are not precursors of more serious TMJ problems (Just et al., 1991).

Question 5, "Orthodontics is the best treatment for TMD in patients with skeletal malocclusion", had 92% disagreement with the consensus. The Manaus and Brasilia samples agreed with the consensus, while the other studies obtained statistically different results. The Kansas and Seattle clinicians were only 28% in disagreement, which may show a very occlusionist view of TMD treatment. Authors confirm the opinion of the experts, disagreeing and saying that orthodontics does not prevent TMD, nor does it cure or treat it (Just et al., 1991; Luther, 1998a; McNamara Jr., 1997; Kim et al., 2002; Machado et al., 2010).

Question 6, "TMD caused by trauma is much more difficult to treat and has a much worse prognosis than other types of TMD", was answered by 85% of the experts, disagreeing with the results of all the other studies. Manaus, on the other hand, agreed with this item by 48%.

Question 7, "transcranial radiography is the most accurate method for visualizing the TMJ" was disagreed with by 77% of the experts, which is surprising since magnetic resonance imaging is the exam of choice for visualizing the TMJ, and transcranial radiography provides a poor image, full of distortions and overlaps, and because it is radiation, it does not allow visualization of soft tissue (Just et al., 1991). The majority of manauaras also disagreed with this item, however, in Kansas and the Seattle Clinicians, there was less than half disagreement. Perhaps this result is a false negative, because in the 1990s, when the questionnaires were administered in the studies prior to those in Manaus and Brasilia, magnetic resonance imaging was not as popular as it is today.

Next, the respondents evaluated two statements about CT scans: "the presence of joint alterations on CT scans together with crepitus in the joints indicates the need for treatment" and "the position of the condyle in the fossa seen on a CT scan is an accurate indicator of joint derangement". The experts disagreed with these statements by 77% and 92% respectively, corroborating the literature, i.e. only the signs and symptoms of TMD that bother the patient such as pain, audible clicks, tinnitus and ear fullness should be treated. Morphological findings that deviate from normality may indicate organic adaptations and not the etiology of the disease (McNeill, 1997a). However, despite this consensus, the sample from Amazonas and the other studies seem to believe that the image is sovereign over the patient's signs and symptoms, as 50% of the experts disagreed with the statement and 25.5% were neutral for the first item and only 40.8% disagreed for the second. The dentists from Brasilia and the specialists from Seattle had the closest disagreements to the experts, with 60.9 and 66.9%, respectively, for the second item.

On question 10, "inferior repositioning plates are more effective than superior plates", 92% of the experts disagreed. The result that was closest to this was achieved in Brasilia with 59.4%, followed by Manaus with 57.1%, which were statistically similar. In the other studies, disagreement was less than 50%. Perhaps the question should be: are repositioning plates effective in treating TMD? McNeill (1997b) reported that plates of some kind have been used to relieve the signs and symptoms of TMD since the beginning of the 20th century. Authors believe that they have some benefit but evidence is lacking (Forsell, Kalso, 2004; Glass et al., 1993). It may be that its benefits are more related to proprioception and placebo than structural changes (McNeill, 1997b).

Question 11, "nocturnal bruxism is caused by occlusal interferences", was where the Amazonian orthodontists most agreed with the consensus, with 73.5% from Manaus against 85% of the consensus who disagreed with this statement. This result is statistically similar to that of Brasilia and different from other studies. It seems that this myth is being overturned.

On the last two pathophysiology questions, there was unanimous agreement among the experts, "cold and/or heat followed by passive muscle stretching are good initial treatments for TMD" and disagreement for "all individuals with TMJ clicks need treatment". In the former, only 61.2% agreed in Manaus, with the Seoul sample, at 75%, coming closest to the experts. It is important to disseminate this information, as it is a simple measure for patients to adopt and can relieve their signs and symptoms while they are waiting to see a TMD/OFD specialist (Medlicott, Harris, 2006; McNeill, 1997b). In the second sentence, the respondents from Kansas and Seattle had statistically similar results to the experts. The Manaus sample disagreed by only 64.3%. This is a low rate, since the need for treatment in the case of TMD must be defined by the patient and their symptoms.

It can therefore be seen that the sample of dentists in Manaus is still unaware of biomedical and biomechanical aspects linked to the etiology, diagnosis and treatment of TMD. Factors such as occlusion and its balance, orthodontic treatment, trauma, repositioning plates and conservative treatments for TMD are a consensus among experts in the field, but seem to be unknown to the majority of the sample studied.

Thus, it could be seen that the pathophysiology of TMD was not yet fully understood by the sample surveyed in Manaus. These results are similar to those found in Seattle (Le Resche et al., 1993), Kansas (Glaros et al., 1994), Seoul (Lee et al., 2000) and Brasilia (Ribeiro, 2009).

6.3.2 Psychophysiology

This area of the questionnaire contains nine items related to the interaction of physical and psychological factors in the etiology, diagnosis and treatment of TMD. Graph 6 shows the frequency distribution of the responses of the Amazonians to the psychophysiology questions, Table 3 compares the responses of the expert consensus with other studies and Graphs 22 to 30 show the responses individually analyzed.

In the very first item, we find the first controversy, because in the statement "the mechanisms of acute and chronic pain are the same", while the consensus unanimously disagreed, Manaus disagreed with 72.4%, a result statistically similar to that of the other cities except Brasilia, which disagreed with 87% of the interviewees. This result is easily justified by the fact that in specialization courses in orthodontics and functional jaw orthopedics, as well as in undergraduate dentistry courses, the subject of "pain" is neither discussed nor addressed in any discipline.

In the second item, "biofeedback" can be useful in the treatment of TMD, it seems that orthodontists in Manaus are unaware of this device since 8 of the 98 interviewees did not answer the question, and of the respondents only 43.9% agreed, with a consensus of 77% agreeing. Both Brasilia, Kansas and Seoul had statistically similar results to Manaus. Medlicott & Harris (2006) said that relaxation and biofeedback techniques can be more effective than occlusal plates.

On item 3, "parafunctional habits are often important in the development of TMD", there was almost a consensus among all the samples, since they all agreed with this statement, with the Manaus sample coming closest to the 85% of experts with 84.7%.

Item 4, "patients who grind and/or clench their teeth do so during the day or night, never both", is incorrect according to the experts (92%). Manaus agreed with the experts and with all the other studies, except for Seoul, where the 57.5% was statistically different from the 74.5% in Manaus. This information is important since one of the main causes of muscular TMD is clenching at night and/or during the day.

Items 5, 6 and 7 address stress as an etiological, precipitating or perpetuating agent of TMD. Item 5, "stress control is indicated for many TMD patients", was unanimous among the experts, with all the samples agreeing except for Seoul, where only 59.5% agreed. In item 6 "stress is the main factor in the development of TMD", 85% of the experts agreed and Manaus and Brasilia agreed with 39.8 and 37.7% respectively. There was some doubt among the Amazonians, and there should be no doubt about this statement, since it is widely believed that stress is an aggravating and perpetuating factor in TMD (McNeill, 1997b; Medlicott, Harris, 2006). And in statement 7, "tension and stress increase the activity of the masticatory muscles in susceptible patients", there was unanimous agreement between the experts, and agreement between the Manaus and Brasilia samples, with results statistically similar to theirs, but different from Seattle, Kansas and Seoul. However, the answer given to the previous item does not demonstrate the knowledge shown by this assertion.

In item 8, "progressive muscle relaxation is not an effective treatment for TMD", it would be reasonable to believe that there would be a high level of disagreement, as there was with 85% of the experts, because if tension and stress increase muscle activity, relaxing these muscles would be a form of treatment for TMD. However, the Manaus respondents disagreed by only 58.2% and all the surveys followed the Manaus trend, except for Seoul, which disagreed by 74%. Could it be that they don't associate TMD with the muscles of mastication?

Item 9, "information on the daily pattern of TMD symptoms may be useful in identifying contributing factors", was agreed upon by all the studies in the 88 to 92% range, except for Seoul, which resulted in only 69% agreement. All case histories for pain are essential as a diagnostic aid.

In general, Manaus had statistically different answers from the consensus in only three items, 1, 2 and 6. In this part of the questionnaire, it was noted that the sample surveyed also recognizes non-occlusal factors in the etiology and development of TMD. The items that mention elements such as parafunctional habits, clenching and bruxism in the development of the problem received high levels of agreement. The available literature recognizes the multifactorial nature of TMD.

TMD and its link to psychological factors (McNeill, 1997b; Carlsson, 2001). Thus, the responses obtained from orthodontists in Amazonas suggest that these professionals are aware of some of the physical and psychological factors related to TMD; however, they need to relate TMD more closely to muscular factors.

6.3.3 Chronic Pain

The Manaus respondents need to improve their knowledge of chronic pain, drug treatment for TMD, surgical indication for TMD, and the interaction between TMD and psychology. All the answers were statistically different (p-value <0.001), except for item 7, which states that "difficulty sleeping is a common finding in chronic pain", where the Manaus sample agreed by 75% and the experts by 96%.

Graph 7 shows the distribution of the frequencies of the answers given by the Amazonians to the chronic pain questions, Table 5 compares the answers of the expert consensus with the other studies and Graphs 31 to 39 show the answers analyzed individually.

In the first statement, "patients with chronic TMD should be advised to rest and limit professional and social activities when in pain", while 85% of the experts disagreed, 50.4% of the Amazonians agreed.

In the statements about the use of medication, there was a low level of agreement between the Amazonians and the experts. In the item "narcotics (as "necessary" for pain) are the treatment of choice when TMD pain is severe", while 93% of the experts disagreed, 53.1% of the Amazonians agreed. With regard to the statement "antidepressants are never indicated in the control of TMD", there was an improvement in the position of the interviewees from Manaus, as they disagreed with the statement with 54.1% while the consensus disagreed with 89%. Perhaps this low level of agreement with the experts indicates a belief on the part of the people of Amazonas regarding the use of medication in the treatment of TMD. Pharmacology is certainly a treatment modality for TMD, but it has been used very little by specialists in the field (Michelotti, Iodice, 2010). In the study by Tegelberg et al. (2001), of the 285 dentists interviewed, only 20 used this method and none of them used it as their first choice of treatment.

The statement assessing knowledge about surgical indication for TMD, "an extensive history of failed treatments for TMD is a common indication for surgery", generated doubt in the Manaus sample, as 43.9% agreed, 30.6% disagreed and 23.5% were neutral, while the experts disagreed 100%. The literature still shows controversy in the treatment of TMD, but there seems to be a consensus among researchers that the treatment of choice should be conservative and reversible (McNeill, 1997b; Carlsson, 2001; Wright, Sluka, 2001; Medlicott, Harris, 2006).

On the questions relating psychology to TMD, the Amazonian sample also disagreed with the experts. The biggest disagreement was with the item that says "chronic pain is a behavioral problem as well as a physical one", since 96% of the experts agreed and 33.7% disagreed. On the other side of the statistics, the answer that came closest to that of the experts was for item 9, "treatment with behavior modification is indicated for patients with chronic painful TMD", since the Manaus orthodontists agreed with 63.3% and the experts 89%. Researchers suggest increasing these activities in order to prevent the development of chronic disabling pain behavior (Le Resche et al.,

1993)

In item 7 "difficulty sleeping is a common finding in chronic pain" there was a statistically similar result in all the samples, including the experts, where everyone agreed in the majority and the closest to 96% of the experts was Kansas with 79% followed by Manaus with 75.5%.

Items 8 and 9 showed more heterogeneous responses between the samples. Question 8 "some patients use pain as an excuse to avoid unpleasant tasks" was agreed upon by the expert consensus with 89% while Manaus, Brasilia, Kansas and Seoul agreed to a lesser extent, with 51%, 57.2%, 61% and 64.5% respectively, statistically different from the Seattle sample. The responses to item 9 "behavior modification treatment is indicated for patients with chronic painful TMD" had a similar distribution to the previous item, i.e. the consensus agreed at 89% and Manaus, Brasilia, Kansas and Seoul agreed to a lesser extent, with 63.3%, 71%, 67% and 64.5% respectively, statistically different from the Seattle sample. Researchers suggest increasing daily activities in order to avoid the development of chronic disabling pain behavior (Le Resche et al., 1993).

Therefore, the statistical analysis showed differences in the responses of the Manaus interviewees and the experts, as mentioned above. These results are similar to those in Brasilia and different to those found in the Seattle, Kansas and Seoul studies, which had results closer to consensus than those in Manaus. Respondents need to improve their knowledge of chronic pain, TMD drug treatment and surgical indications for TMD treatment. All the answers were statistically different (p-value <0.005) from the experts except one.

6.3.4 Psychiatric disorders

This part consisted of four items relating anxiety, depression and somatization commonly associated with TMD. Most of the interviewees agreed with the experts on all the items, demonstrating knowledge of the relationship between psychiatric factors and TMD.

The responses of the dentists in the Manaus sample showed agreement with the experts on the items about the involvement of psychiatric disorders with TMD, except for the statement "Clinical depression is rare in patients with chronic TMD", where the experts disagreed 100% and Manaus disagreed 62.2%.

Graph 8 shows the distribution of the frequencies of responses on the subject of Psychiatric Disorders, Table 7 compares the consensus of the experts with the responses of the professionals in the samples studied and Graphs 40 to 43 show each response individually analyzed.

In the items stating that "depressive behavior is common in TMD patients", "anxiety disorders are more common in TMD patients than in the general population" and "depression can be an important etiological factor in chronic pain", the results were statistically similar to those of the experts and the other samples, since the p-values were above 0.005, with the exception of the last one, which was different only in the Kansas and Seattle samples.

It should be noted that the dentists surveyed recognize that anxiety and depressive behavior are common in TMD patients, endorsing research which cites that TMD rarely occurs alone (McNeill, 1997a) and, therefore, treatment should be multidisciplinary and multiaxial, also involving psychology and psychiatry professionals (McNeill, 1997b; Venâncio, Camparis, 2002). Therefore, dentists should recognize and refer TMD patients for the necessary follow-up (Glaros et al., 1994; McNeill, 1997b).

6.4 Final considerations

Looking at all the data collected and discussed, it is clear that there is a large gap between the consensus of professionals who research and produce scientific material on TMD and the opinions of orthodontists in Manaus on some of the topics covered. The answers to each item can be analyzed as a reflection of the professionals' academic training combined with their clinical experience and professional retraining. Thus, it can be seen that researchers in the field have a clearer vision and fewer uncertainties on the subject, so much so that a consensus has been formed among them. On the other hand, the responses from the Manaus sample show uncertainty about various aspects of TMD and disagreement with the researchers in the field. At this point, there is a significant difference between scientific knowledge and clinical practice.

Just et al., 1991, came to a similar conclusion: although research has led to a better understanding of the cause, diagnosis and treatment of TMD, the large discrepancy between the scientific literature and the opinions presented in the study represents a general lack of knowledge about some of the research carried out in the last 10 years in the area of temporomandibular disorders.

Knowing that knowledge is dynamic and that at any moment what was believed at the beginning of the 1990s can be changed by clinical evidence, it can be asked whether the experts' answers at that time would still be the same if they were questioned today. The answer is yes, as explained below.

Tegelberg et al. (2007) used a questionnaire to **assess** dentists' knowledge of TMD in children and adolescents in Sweden. The answers to the questionnaire were given by 19 TMD specialists who had documented research activity and were members of the Swedish Academy of Temporomandibular Disorders.

The questionnaire contained 37 statements about etiology, diagnosis, classification, chronic pain and pain behavior, treatment and prognosis. Each statement was judged on a 0-10 point scale with the terminal definitions agree or disagree. This questionnaire was based on that of the University of Washington in Seattle, with some minor modifications to direct the research towards dentists' knowledge of temporomandibular disorders in children and adolescents.

Of the 37 statements, 20 were contained in the Washington questionnaire, and although there were points with statistically different answers, there was no disagreement on any of the items between the experts in Sweden and those in Washington. This may show that over 15 years, the knowledge about TMD contained in the questionnaires has not changed.

We may be heading towards a single truth about TMD. However, this truth must be disseminated and reach all DCs who treat TMD, and orthodontists are still highly sought-after specialists and referrers for the treatment of this disorder, who need to understand and know the subject well in order to conduct proper treatment and control of this condition.

Perhaps a practical way to make knowledge arrive more quickly would be to include the subject of TMD/OFD in the syllabuses and menus of some undergraduate and postgraduate courses in orthodontics, or even as a subject, since it became a specialty 12 years ago. Only in this way, with trained professionals, will we be able to control our patients' TMD properly.

7 CONCLUSION

Considering the data discussed, it can be concluded that:

a) The knowledge of orthodontists and/or functional jaw orthopedists in Amazonas matches that of the other samples compared in this study and disagrees with the experts on several items, especially in the area of TMD-related chronic pain, followed by the areas of psychophysiology, pathophysiology and psychiatric disorders.

8 REFERENCES [1]

Baharvand M, Monfared MS, Hamian M, Moghaddam EJ, Hosseini FS, Alavi K. Temporomandibular disorders: knowledge, attitude and practice among dentists in Tehran, Iran. Journal of dental research, dental clinics, dental prospects. 2010; 4(3):90- 4.

Carlsson GE. Critical commentary 1: the etipology of temporomandibular disorder: implication for treatment. J Orofac Pain. 2001;15:106-8.

Carlsson GE, Magnusson T, Guimaraes AS. Treatment of temporomandibular disorders in the dental clinic. Sao Paulo: Quintessence; 2006.

Casagrande E, Rossato C. The relationship between orthodontic treatment and temporomandibular disorder. Ortodontia. 1998, Jan/Feb; 31(1): 80-7.

Francesquini Jr L, Francesquini MA, Daruge E, Gonçalves RJ, Ambrosano GMB, Rizatti Barbosa CM. TMJ dysfunction - verification of dental surgeons' knowledge of etiology, incidence and diagnosis. JBO. 1999, 4(19):68-79.

Forssell H, Kalso E, Koskela P, Vehmanen R, Puukka P, Alanen P. Occlusal treatments in temporomandibular disorders: a qualitative systematic review of randomized controlled trials. Pain. 1999; 83(3): 549-60

Forssell H, Kalso E. Application of principles of evidence-based medicine to occlusal treatments for temporomandibular disorders: are there lessons to be learned? J Orofac Pain. 2004; 18(1):9-22.

Glaros AG, Glass EG, McLaughlin L. Knowledge and beliefs of dentists regarding temporomandibular disorders and chronic pain. J Orofac Pain. 1994; 8(2):216-222.

Glass EG, Glaros AG, McGlynn FD. Myofascial pain dysfunction: treatments used by ADA members. Cranio, 1993, Jan; 11(1):25-29.

Grossmann E, Grossmann TK. Temporomandibular joint surgery. Rev Dor. 2011, Apr-Jun;12(2):152-9

Just JK; Perry HT, Greene CS. Treating TM disorders: a survey on diagnosis, etiology and management. J Am Dent Assoc, 1991; 122(9):55-60

Kim MR, Graber TM, Viana MA. Orthodontics and temporomandibular disorder: a metaanalysis. Am J Orthod Dentofacial Orthop. 2002, May;121(5):438-46.

According to the Standardization Manual for Dissertations and Theses of the CPO Sao Leopoldo Mandic Postgraduate Center, based on the 2007 Vancouver style, and abbreviation of journal titles in accordance with Index Medicus.

Lee WY, Choi JW, Lee JW. A study of dentists' knowledge and beliefs regarding temporomandibular disorders in Korea. Cranio. 2000 Apr;18(2):142-6.

Le Resche L, Truelove EL, Dworkin S. Temporomandibular disorder: a survey of dentist's knowledge and beliefs. J Am Dent Assoc. 1993; 124(5):90-106.

Luther, F. Orthodontics and the temporomandibular joint: where are we now? Part 1: Orthodontic treatment and temporomandibular disorders. Angle Orthod. 1998a, August; . 68(4):295-304.

Luther, F. Orthodontics and the temporomandibular joint: where are we now? Part 2. Functional occlusion, malocclusion, and TMD. Angle Orthod. 1998b, August; 68(4):305- 18.

Machado E, Machado P, Cunali PA, Grehs RA. Orthodontics as risk factor for temporomandibular disorders : a systematic review. Dental Press J Orthod. 2010; 15(5): 174-83.

Manfredi AP, Silva AA, Vendite LL. Evaluation of the sensitivity of the screening questionnaire for orofacial pain and temporomandibular disorders recommended by the American Academy of Orofacial Pain. Rev Bras Otorrinolaringol. 2001; 67(6):763-8.

Mao, Y.; Duan, X. H. Attitude of Chinese orthodontists towards the relationship between orthodontic treatment and temporomandibular disorders. Int Dent Journal.2001, August; 51(4):277-81.

McNamara Jr. JA. Orthodontic treatment and temporomandibular disorders. Oral Surg Oral Med Oral Pathol Oral Radiol Endod.1997, Jan; 83(1):107-17.

McNeill, C. History and evolution of TMD concepts. Oral surgery, oral medicine, oral pathology, oral radiology, and endodontics. 1997a; 83(1):51-60

McNeill, C. Management of temporomandibular disorders: concepts and controversies.

The Journal of prosthetic dentistry. 1997b; 77(5):510-22

Medlicott MS; Harris SR. Research report: A systematic review of the effectiveness of exercise , manual therapy , electrotherapy , relaxation training , and biofeedback in the management of temporomandibular disorder. Physical Therapy. 2006 86(7):956-73

Michelotti A, Iodice G. The role of orthodontics in temporomandibular disorders. Journal of oral rehabilitation. 2010; 37(6): 411-29.

Moana Filho EJ. Survey of orthodontists' attitudes and beliefs regarding temporomandibular dysfunction and orofacial pain. Dental Press Journal of Orthodontics and Facial Orthopedics. 2005; 10(4):60-75.

Mohl ND, Ohrbach R. The dilemma of scientific knowledge versus clinical management of temporomandibular disorder. J Prosthet Dent. 1992;67:11-20.

Parashos P, Morgan MV, Messer HH. Response rate and nonresponse bias in a questionnaire survey of dentists. Community Dental Oral Epidemiol. 2005;33:9-16.

Tegelberg A, List T, Wahlund K, Wenneberg B. Temporomandibular disorders in children and adolescents: a survey of dentists' attitudes, routine and experience. Swedish Dental Journal. 2001;

25(3): 119-27.

Tegelberg A, Wenneberg B, List T. General practice dentists' knowledge of temporomandibular disorders in children and adolescents. European Journal of Dental Education. 2007; 11(3):216-21.

Ribeiro VP. Evaluation of the knowledge of dental surgeons in Brasilia about the area of temporomandibular dysfunction [dissertation]. Campinas: Sao Leopoldo Mandic Postgraduate Center; 2009.

Venâncio R, Camparis C. Temporomandibular disorders: a study of the procedures performed by professionals. Rev Odontol UNESP. 2002;31(2):191-203.

Wright A, Sluka KA. Nonpharmacological treatments for musculoskeletal pain. Clin J Pain. 2001;17(1):33-46.

9 ANNEXES

ANNEX A - Project Approval Sheet

São Leopoldo Mandic
Faculdade de Odontologia
Centro de Pesquisas Odontológicas
Certificado de Cumprimento de Princípios Éticos

C E R T I F I C O que, após analisar o projeto de pesquisa

Título *Conhecimento dos Ortodontistas do Estado do Amazonas a Respeito de Disfunção Temporomandibular e Dor Orofacial*

Pesquisador principal: Heráclio Alves Barbosa Júnior

Orientador: Antônio Sérgio Guimarães

Data Avaliação: 4/4/2011   Nº Protocolo: 2011/0032

o Comitê de Ética em Pesquisa (CEP) da Faculdade de Odontologia e Centro de Pesquisas Odontológicas São Leopoldo Mandic considerou que o projeto está de acordo com as diretrizes para a proteção do sujeito de pesquisa, estabelecidas pela Resolução nº 196/96, do Conselho Nacional de Saúde, do Ministério da Saúde.

Campinas, SP, Brazil,   quarta-feira, 6 de abril de 2011

- - - - - - - - - - - - - - - -

CERTIFICATION OF COMPLIANCE WITH ETHICAL PRINCIPLES

I hereby, certify that upon analysis of the Research Project,

Title: Amazonas State Orthodontists' Knowledge Concerning Temporomandibular Disorders and Orofacial Pain

Main Researcher(Author):   Heráclio Alves Barbosa Júnior

Advisor: Antônio Sérgio Guimarães

the Committee of Ethics for Research of São Leopoldo Mandic School of Dentistry and Research Center, has considered the mentioned project to be in accordance to the guidelines of protection to the subject of the research, established by the Regulation number 196/96, from the National Health Council of the Brazilian Health Ministry.

Profa. Dra. Sônia Vieira
Presidente do Comitê de Ética e Pesquisa

070873

INFORMED CONSENT FORM

I'm studying Amazonas orthodontists' knowledge of Temporomandibular Dysfunction (TMD) and Orofacial Pain.

If you agree to take part in this research, which will be my master's thesis, please fill in the attached questionnaire, which consists of some professional data and statements followed by a numerical scale between "I TOTALLY DISAGREE" and "I TOTALLY AGREE" about the diagnosis and treatment of TMD. All the statements must be answered by ticking only one option.

Your participation is not obligatory, but if you decide to cooperate, all the information will be used in statistical studies and your data will remain confidential. You are also guaranteed the freedom to refuse or withdraw consent without penalty.

If you have any questions or comments about the questionnaire or the dissertation, please contact: e-mail xxxxxxxxxxxx; telephone (xx)xxxx xxxx (office hours) or (xx) xxxx xxxx.

Thank you for your cooperation.

Sincerely.

Heraclio Alves Barbosa Junior CRO-AM 1545

I declare that I agree to participate in Dr. Heràclio Alves Barbosa Junior's research of my own free will, without any expense on my part and without any kind of payment for this participation:

NAME: ________________________________RG: _____________ DATE: __/__/___

STUDY ON

DENTAL SURGEONS' KNOWLEDGE OF

TEMPOROMANDIBULAR DISORDERS

GUIDELINES:

1. Each statement is followed by a scale ranging from TOTALLY DISAGREE to TOTALLY AGREE.

2. Read and evaluate each statement according to YOUR KNOWLEDGE OR OPINION.

3. Mark with an "X" only ONE value for each statement.

4. Fill in ALL the fields and answer ALL the questions.

QUESTIONNAIRE

AGE: GENDER: MF ˌYEAR OF GRADUATION:

SPECIALTY(S) COMPLETED ____

YEAR OF COMPLETION OF THE SPECIALIZATION COURSE(S):_____________

DO YOU WORK IN AMAZONAS? YES NO

1 PATHOPHYSIOLOGY

1) Interference on the non-working side (balance) is commonly related to TMD.

TOTALLY DISAGREE	0 1 2 3 4 5 6 7 8 9 10	TOTALLY AGREE

2. Balancing occlusion is an early treatment for TMD.

TOTALLY DISAGREE	0 1 2 3 4 5 6 7 8 9 10	TOTALLY AGREE

3. Orthodontic treatment can prevent the onset of TMD.

TOTALLY DISAGREE	0 1 2 3 4 5 6 7 8 9 10	TOTALLY AGREE

4. Surgical arthroscopy is almost completely effective in repositioning the disc in cases of internal joint disruption.

TOTALLY DISAGREE	0 1 2 3 4 5 6 7 8 9 10	TOTALLY AGREE

5. Orthodontics is the best treatment for TMD in patients with skeletal malocclusion.

TOTALLY DISAGREE	0 1 2 3 4 5 6 7 8 9 10	TOTALLY AGREE

6. TMD caused by trauma is much more difficult to treat and has a much worse prognosis than other types of TMD. ____

TOTALLY DISAGREE	0	1	2	3	4	5	6	7	8	9	10	TOTALLY AGREE

7. Transcranial radiography is the most accurate method of visualizing the TMJ.

TOTALLY DISAGREE	0	1	2	3	4	5	6	7	8	9	10	TOTALLY AGREE

8. The presence of joint changes on CT scans together with crepitus in the joints indicates the need for treatment.____

TOTALLY DISAGREE	0	1	2	3	4	5	6	7	8	9	10	TOTALLY AGREE

9. The position of the condyle in the fossa seen on a CT scan is an accurate indicator of joint disruption.

TOTALLY DISAGREE	0	1	2	3	4	5	6	7	8	9	10	TOTALLY AGREE

10. Lower repositioning plates are more effective than upper plates.

TOTALLY DISAGREE	0	1	2	3	4	5	6	7	8	9	10	TOTALLY AGREE

11. Night bruxism is caused by occlusal interference.

TOTALLY DISAGREE	0	1	2	3	4	5	6	7	8	9	10	TOTALLY AGREE

12. Cold and/or heat followed by passive muscle stretching are good initial treatments for TMD.

TOTALLY DISAGREE	0	1	2	3	4	5	6	7	8	9	10	TOTALLY AGREE

13. All individuals with TMJ clicks need treatment.

TOTALLY DISAGREE	0	1	2	3	4	5	6	7	8	9	10	TOTALLY AGREE

2 PSYCHOPHYSIOLOGY:

1. The mechanisms of acute and chronic pain are the same.

TOTALLY DISAGREE	0	1	2	3	4	5	6	7	8	9	10	TOTALLY AGREE

2. biofeedback can be useful in the treatment of TMD.

TOTALLY DISAGREE	0	1	2	3	4	5	6	7	8	9	10	TOTALLY AGREE

3. Parafunctional habits are often important in the development of TMD.

TOTALLY DISAGREE	0	1	2	3	4	5	6	7	8	9	10	TOTALLY AGREE

4. Patients who grind and/or clench their teeth do so during the day or night, never both.

TOTALLY DISAGREE	0	1	2	3	4	5	6	7	8	9	10	TOTALLY AGREE

5. Stress management is indicated for many TMD patients.

TOTALLY DISAGREE	0	1	2	3	4	5	6	7	8	9	10	TOTALLY AGREE

6. Stress is the main factor in the development of TMD.

TOTALLY DISAGREE	0	1	2	3	4	5	6	7	8	9	10	TOTALLY AGREE

7. Tension and stress increase the activity of the masticatory muscles in susceptible patients.

TOTALLY DISAGREE	0	1	2	3	4	5	6	7	8	9	10	TOTALLY AGREE

8. Muscle relaxation proc resilient is not ra effective treatment for TMD.

TOTALLY DISAGREE	0	1	2	3	4	5	6	7	8	9	10	TOTALLY AGREE

9. Information on the daily pattern of TMD symptoms can be useful in identifying contributing factors.

TOTALLY DISAGREE	0	1	2	3	4	5	6	7	8	9	10	TOTALLY AGREE

3 CHRONIC PAIN:

1. Patients with chronic TMD should be advised to rest and limit professional and social activities when in pain.

TOTALLY DISAGREE	0	1	2	3	4	5	6	7	8	9	10	TOTALLY AGREE

2. Narcotics (as "necessaries" for pain) are the treatment of choice when TMD pain is severe.

TOTALLY DISAGREE	0	1	2	3	4	5	6	7	8	9	10	TOTALLY AGREE

3. Antidepressants are never indicated in the control of TMD.

TOTALLY DISAGREE	0	1	2	3	4	5	6	7	8	9	10	TOTALLY AGREE

4. An extensive history of failed treatments for TMD is a common indication for surgery.

TOTALLY DISAGREE	0	1	2	3	4	5	6	7	8	9	10	TOTALLY AGREE

5. Chronic pain is a behavioral problem as well as a physical one.

TOTALLY DISAGREE	0	1	2	3	4	5	6	7	8	9	10	TOTALLY AGREE

6. Although some TMD patients have psychological problems, these are usually not related to pain.

TOTALLY DISAGREE	0	1	2	3	4	5	6	7	8	9	10	TOTALLY AGREE

7. Difficulty sleeping is a common finding in chronic pain.

TOTALLY DISAGREE	0	1	2	3	4	5	6	7	8	9	10	TOTALLY AGREE

8. Some patients use pain as an excuse to avoid unpleasant tasks.

TOTALLY DISAGREE	0	1	2	3	4	5	6	7	8	9	10	TOTALLY AGREE

9. Behavior modification treatment is indicated for patients with chronic painful TMD.

TOTALLY DISAGREE	0	1	2	3	4	5	6	7	8	9	10	TOTALLY AGREE

4 PSYCHIATRIC DISORDERS:

1. Clinical depression is rare in patients with chronic TMD.

TOTALLY DISAGREE	0	1	2	3	4	5	6	7	8	9	10	TOTALLY AGREE

2. Depressive behavior is common in TMD patients.

TOTALLY DISAGREE	0	1	2	3	4	5	6	7	8	9	10	TOTALLY AGREE

3. Anxiety disorders are more common in TMD patients than in the general population.

TOTALLY DISAGREE	0	1	2	3	4	5	6	7	8	9	10	TOTALLY AGREE

4. Depression can be an important etiological factor in chronic pain.

TOTALLY DISAGREE	0	1	2	3	4	5	6	7	8	9	10	TOTALLY AGREE

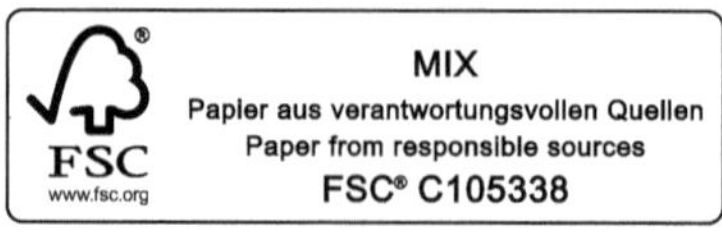

Printed by Books on Demand GmbH, Norderstedt / Germany